Self-Reliance
The Future of Child Health and Development

A Volume in the *Iketsetseng* Series
For the Health and Welfare of Children

What is the *Iketsetseng* Series?

This book is a fourth volume in the experimental *Iketsetseng* series. *Iketsetseng* is a word from Lesotho meaning, roughly, "do it yourselves". The Symbol of the series is a small deer, Sang Kancil, from Malaysia. This deer is renowned for its ability to get on in the jungle, to be self-reliant, and to take the appropriate initiatives to extract itself from difficult situations. It is also the name of a self-reliant project in the urban squatter settlements of Kuala Lumpur.

This experimental series presents ideas to promote the health and welfare of children. It is intended as a means of encouraging exchanges of views about health and development ideas that may lead to, and reflect, more effective action to combat poverty, deprivation and exploitation.

Iketsetseng documents are contibutions to continuing conversations amongst those who care for, and are concerned with, the health and welfare of children. Each action book focuses on a specific problem and proposes a number of specific solutions involving the maximum of self-reliance. They are the cooperative efforts of authors from many countries, all with a first-hand knowledge of poverty situations. The aim is to reflect and to promote the ideas of the communities themselves. Indeed it is hoped that ways can be found of giving people themselves a forum to express their needs and opinions.

The *Iketsetseng* papers are not offical policy documents in any sense, but should stimulate more critical thinking which will in turn lead to more effective policies and actions. Designed to bring useful ideas out into the open, these publications are in no way definitive but will hopefully lead, after fuller dialogue, to more comprehensive works and more effective action. Useful comments will also be published.

This series originated as part of a cooperative programme between the World Health Organisation and the Swedish Government agencies (SIDA-SAREC).

Self-Reliance

The Future of Child Health and Development

Sponsored by
Defence for Children International, Geneva

Mouton Publishers
Berlin · New York · Amsterdam

ISBN 90 279 3390 1 (cloth edition)
90 279 3400 2 (paper edition)

 Printing: Druckerei Hildebrand, Berlin . — Binding: Lüderitz & Bauer Buchgewerbe GmbH, Berlin. — Coverphoto by Ullstein, Berlin.
Printed in Germany

Contents

About the Sponsor for this Volume

The Defence for Children International Movement is an independent, non-govermental organisation set up during the International Year of the Child (1979) and based in Geneva, Switzerland. Its purposes are to respond - on request or on its own initiative - to individual and group situations in which the fundamental rights of the child are deemed to be violated, and to carry out international advocacy on the issues involved in order to prevent such violations, to promote the practical observance of children's rights, and to arouse awareness at all levels regarding neglect or violation of these rights.

Its work is financed by grants from international and national bodies, both governmental and non-governmental, foundations and — being a movement — by the membership dues of its individual and organisational affiliates.

Defence for Children International's sponsorship of publications in the *Iketsetseng* series comes within its preventive advocacy and conscientisation activity.

Defence for Children International is the only international action agency specifically and solely concerned with the protection of children's rights. For more information on its overall work, please contact:

Defence for Children International
P.O. Box 92
CH-1226 GENEVA-THONEX

CHAPTER ONE

WHAT HAPPENED AT SHANGHAI

Introduced here is the theme of more effective community action in maternal and child health as a major intersectoral contribution to development from below. It is based on a paper which emerged from the discussions and deliberations of a group of MCH workers from a wide variety of countries who met together under WHO auspices in Shanghai in June 1980.

1. THE WELLBEING OF WOMEN AND CHILDREN AND DEVELOPMENT

The goal of health for all by the year 2000 is one to which all nations of the world have subscribed, but there are doubts whether present approaches will lead there. And in no area is this more true than in maternal and child health.

In the industrialized, but particularly in the non-industrialized countries women and children are exposed to greater health and social risks than others. Their needs, problems and aspirations have been unrecognized and unacknowledged.

Sickness and death rates are high, and social opportunity is limited, both major factors in retarding socioeconomic development. Health and socioeconomic development are deeply related movements, and the wellbeing of women and children are essential to both.

2. INVOLVING COMMUNITIES

How to initiate and maintain the momentum for women and children remains a vital question. Many of the approaches that have been developed and tried in the past, especially in the field of health care, have shown a singular inability to reach those at greatest risk, or to meet the full range of needs of those who have been reached. Health care services have often contradicted local customs and expectations, failing to build upon the resources of communities and in so doing have reduced any effectiveness they might have had. All too rarely have communities been involved, together with the health care system, in identifying problems, establishing priorities, or in planning and implementing appropriate strategies to meet them. The relationship of many health care systems to the community has been a socially distant one of a provider/client nature.

In many settings, the health care systems are unable or unwilling to adapt quickly enough. Much more account has to be taken of the character of communities, their expectations, their needs and possibilities. The community must be actively involved at all levels. Any health activity, especially maternal and child health, can be the entry point for the range of development activities.

3. THE BASIC TASKS

What is needed is to identify first of all the fundamental needs and wants of mothers and children. Then it is a question of seeing how community based organizations can best meet these needs and wants, and how the health services can help. What may be needed is a network of maternal and child health workers, drawing from different backgrounds and disciplines, working with other sectors, and facilitating wherever possible; exchanges, ideas and assistance.

4. THE UNIVERSAL NEEDS

The history of health care has time and again demonstrated the broad cultural diversity that exists in the ways in which health and social needs are perceived, and in which priorities are set. But, despite these differences, there remain some universal values and expectations.

a) that every woman should have a healthy pregnancy from which there is a safe outcome for her child

b) that every child should have the opportunities for sound growth and development

c) that every child should have a safe and healthy environment

d) that every child should have adequate social, intellectual and emotional stimulation

e) that every woman should have a life that is socially and emotionally satisfying.

While many of these needs can be met in part through maternal and child health services, the closest collaboration of all sectors is required. The community's participation in all aspects of health and social management, especially at the fundamental planning and implementation stage is a pre-requisite if community needs and wants are to be fulfilled.

5. WHAT SERVICES ARE NEEDED

Below are set out the needs together with the kinds of services that might be developed to help meet them.

Universal needs	Service requirements
Healthy and safe pregnancy and a healthy baby	Early contact and rapport with mother, knowledge about most prevalent complications in pregnancy, safe delivery, sound knowledge of social and cultural contexts e.g. women's work patterns and family life.
Healthy growth and development	Information and trends and practices in child feeding, child rearing and care patterns of growth, regular contact with children and mothers. Information on local trends in the epidemiology of childhood diseases, disabilities, facilities and opportunities for rehabilitation, expectations in community.
Safe and healthy environment	Intersectoral information on health beliefs and behaviour, sources of water and waste disposal habits, community knowledge about relationship between behaviour and environment and disease, regular interaction with community.
Social, intellectual and emotional stimulation for the child	Community and individual resources for caring for children and providing early education, helping motivate communities to participate.

A socially and emotionally satisfying life for women	Involvement of women in planning, close collaboration between the health sector and other sectors that relate to women's daily lives.

6. THE NEED FOR INFORMATION

One of the major themes is the need for information that is reliable, that can be gathered regularly and rapidly, and which accurately reflects the grass-roots situation. While there are various ways in which such data could be obtained, the collection and analysis of community data by the community itself at the grass-roots level is probably the most relevant, efficient and productive. Both in terms of its contribution to planning and evaluation as well as its indirect role in bringing the community into the process of problem assessment and management, local collection of data however simplified and non-specific, can be of much greater value than alternative data collection procedures that rely upon top down, highly technical, often sporadic outside inputs. Certainly, most communities already comment on local production, on employment, on patterns of morbidity and mortality, on the environment, and so on. But often their voices are not heard or listened to, and the genuine individual cries are lost in a welter of anonymous official statistics and processed reports.

7. IDENTIFYING PROBLEMS

Data collection, however, is only one of the activities that communities can undertake as equal partners in the health process. As a first phase in the development of any health care activity, the identification, even if very basic, of health and social problems can and should be undertaken primarily by the community in conjuction with technical personnel.

The potential of the community as an agency for epidemiological work needs to be recognized and built upon; its proximity to problem situations and its understanding of the factors underlying and contributing to them may well prove superior to any analysis undertaken by outside planners less intimately familiar with the situation and less sympathetic to it. In terms of the time and resources involved in such problem identification exercises, diagnoses that are undertaken by the community, or with its close involvement, can represent an appreciable saving and an increase in efficiency.

8. THE NEED FOR THE LOCAL AND THE TRADITIONAL

Again, the identification of acceptable manpower resources, often already selected and acknowledged by local people as sources of health care and advice, represent an especially valuable function. Traditional birth attendants or traditional healers are important sources of community based care and can be readily strengthened to form the springboard for maternal and child health care activities. A traditional practice such as breastfeeding is probably the single, most important element in improving infant health. School teachers, religious leaders, women's groups, local agricultural extension workers similarly all constitute a potential grass-roots base for health activities, and a link and buffer with the outside world. The broader their occupational or sectoral background, and the more contacts they have had with both the community and the outside, the more useful they will be.

9. YOUNG PEOPLE TO THE FORE

In many communities young people are most open to new ideas and able to take on new responsibilities. Their better educational attainments allows them a greater freedom of imagination and insight into problems and possibilities.

They constitute a valuable resource for social change and the development of activities designed to provide support for mothers and children, sensitizing the community to needs and potentials and providing access to relevant information and outside resources.

Much of what is required to improve maternal and child health can be accomplished at the level of the family. For example, a more appropriate division of labour that acknowledges the needs of women as mothers, and rewards more adequately their contribution to the family economy, could do much to bring about better maternal health and through it, better child health. Both in work outside the home and within it, greater sharing of responsibilities between spouses as opposed to the dominant trend of female exploitation can ensure a decreased physical load on the mother and her better physical and mental wellbeing. Sometimes it is a matter of simply getting enough food. Similarly, too many children are exploited at work, and do not receive adequate nutrition in relation to their growth needs and exertions. A better understanding of the needs of women, mothers and children within the family is thus a key priority and should be promoted through every available educational and promotional technique appropriate to the socio-cultural conditions.

10. SELF MANAGEMENT

The task of the community is not only problem identification, data gathering and self help activities. What is also needed at the grass-roots level is a management capability. Ranking of priorities for action, monitoring and evaluation of service activities and back-up provided by other levels of the health care system and other sectors, are integral parts of the health care process that should ideally be in the hands of the community. In many instances this will necessitate the development of new criteria for evaluation, new reporting methods and new channels of communication between the grass-roots level and service administrative levels.

11. THE ROLE OF THE HEALTH CARE SYSTEM AND OTHER SECTORS IN PROMOTING AND SUPPORTING MCH CARE AT THE GRASS-ROOTS LEVEL

Intersectoral collaboration is a sine qua non of grass-roots maternal and child health, but the health care system can often play an instrumental role in initially promoting grass-roots maternal and child health care.

Awareness or identification of local issues, problems and needs has, to be followed by a problem solving phase in which all sectors must participate with the community in seeking the most appropriate and effective ways of dealing with local situations. The consideration of alternative strategies and the selection of the ones most appropriate to local rosources and conditions ideally involves a series of in-depth discussion with those most affected and likely to be involved in following up this phase. Community leaders, womens groups, school teachers, health workers and agricultural agents, for example, should be considered as collaborators. While it may be difficult to involve all the community at all times in these discussions attention should be given to ensuring that the views of all sectors of the community are taken into account, especially those who are most affected by inadequate living conditions and poor health. Community leaders may not always be representative of these groups and there are bound to be conflicts, for which equitable solutions must be found. Community health workers have to be accountable to the community and its delegated authorities.

12. SPECIFIC ROLES FOR THE HEALTH CARE SYSTEM - TASK ANALYSIS

A fundamental aspect of generating new activities and responsibilities is the determination of what different tasks are required and who, under what conditions can effectively perform them. This delineation of tasks, the assessment of existing human resources and identification of required training, requires the technical support of all sectors. Task analysis cannot be undertaken by inexperienced personnel and should be seen as a primary function of the technical support system.

Not only does task analysis permit an assessment of what is required, it alo permits the technical support system to evaluate the feasibility of local programmes and the need for back-up services.

In the area of maternal and child health existing traditional resources and services should be carefully taken into account. The possibilities for additional training of traditional birth attendants and healers for example should be part of the process.

13. SPECIFIC ROLES - TRAINING

The importance of training local manpower, whether in health or other types of work, cannot be underestimated as a contribution to local self-dependence and development. This is especially true if training is undertaken as part of an overall process in which the public has been involved in identifying and assessing problems and has participated closely in proposing the type of action designed to correct those problems.

In the area of maternal and child health care a variety of sectors should be involved in the training process since it is unlikely that any one sector will be able to provide the type of expertise ideally required to prepare the grass-roots workers for the wide range of activities that would ultimately benefit mothers and children.

Training undertaken with the collaboration of different sectors also provides an additional function. It exposes the public as well as the individuals being trained to the network of referral facilities that are available and can be used. This subsequently may be one of the ways in which a continued dialogue can be assured between the community and local and regional government.

Different combinations of training may be required according to the needs of the community and the resources available. As well as the provision of courses for health-related workers, refresher and up-grading training should be made available to local Traditional Birth Attendants and other persons already providing health care, especially where that care has attained a high degree of acceptance and local institutionalisation.

14. SPECIFIC ROLES - DATA COLLECTION

As we have said, a basic part of grass-roots maternal and child health care, as at any other level, is the regular collection and use of relevant data that can be used in the on-going planning, evaluation and prediction of activities and trends.

In the past it has often been assumed that data collection can only be collected reliably by highly trained personnel and at considerable expense. One result has been that poor communities have been overlooked. Alternatively, sophisticated models and approaches have been introduced in circumstances where their cost-effectiveness has been low and where, because the community has not understood the purposes of the data, there has been a weak participation. Conventional recording of vital statistics has often produced unreliable community data; highly complex health record cards which involve extensive time on the part of health staff and patients. These have often gone unutilised simply because of the excessive data items gathered and the confusion incurred through them. The community should therefore not only understand the purposes and value of data, but also that these data be kept simple and essential. Most important is data that can be registered and kept by the family at home. Growth charts or sickness cards, for example, could be designed with this in mind. Family records need not, and should not be limited to health alone but could involve other aspects of family life such as nutrition information, budgeting, environmental needs, and perceptions of the quality of life and development. The different sectors should encourage and be able to record and use "soft data", particularly the wide variety of opinion that people themselves voice. New techniques, such as the delphi method (i.e. putting questions to a range of knowledgeable people) could be used here, but it may be better to build on traditional means of oral or written communications.

15. SPECIFIC ROLES - INTERSECTORAL COOPERATION

Data collection and analysis is also an educational experience and can help make communities conscious of the inter-relationships between environmental, economic, social and other situations and how they affect the health of mothers and children.

The types of information gathered by the community at the grass-roots level will vary in different situations. But it should be easily obtained, relevant to community concerns, and be extracted voluntarily.

Much of the information needed for the organization and improvement of maternal and child care at the grass-roots level is likely to be available through families and much of it may already be known to village leaders, local health workers, etc. and have been gathered in an anecdotal fashion. The task that remains in many situations is to determine what is actually available, what are the sources, and then what are likely to be the most effective ways of drawing that information out and using it on a regular basis.

Mortality data is hard to collect, and much on health and morbidity may be revealed by data from other sectors. In the agricultural sector, for example data on: the types of landholdings and size; types of crops grown (and the ratios of cash and subsistence); seasonality of crops and variation in levels of productivity; market fluctuations in respect to cash cropping; availability of, and need for, technical advisers are all likely to yield insights that influence maternal and child health.

Important education information would be the proportion of children of specific ages who are enrolled and attend school (and the sex ratio), the content of courses offered and especially the relationship to the community situation, environmental hygiene, nutrition, family life, sex education, agriculture, etc. All this would also allow target groups to be identified.

Social support and employment trends are again vital issues in the management of health at the grass-roots level and here the key questions are the availability and cost of creches or day care facilities; technical training and re-training programmes (especially for unemployed); the nature and recipients of maternity leave and allowances: the patterns of work (notably the proportions and those in regular paid employment); the existence of programmes specifically for the protection of women (as for example in China with respect to menstruation, pregnancy, puerperium and lactation); the nature of labour migration (especially sex ratios); the patterns of child care and their relationship to working conditions, etc.

Finally, the data collected by the community should provide a base for the evaluation of local services designed to improve maternal and child health, and the monitoring, of health status itself in the community. The monitoring should build upon existing systems of simple and reliable data gathering and not seek to create new ones. Local personnel should be primarily responsible for the montoring following, wherever possible, existing social networks. There should be a guarantee of a two-way flow of any and all information gathered.

Because health and social development are so closely intertwined, health workers must work closely with other sectors. Equally it should be expected that education, agriculture and public works agents should be prepared to support health personnel in achieving their goals when the community indicates that better health is a felt need.

The determining factor should always be the wishes of the community as expressed in its dialogues with representatives of the different sectors.

Particularly in the case of the health of mothers and children it should be recognised by all concerned that socioeconomic change as represented, for instance by improvements in water supply, fuel gathering, housing and sanitation, work load reducing techniques and more egalitarian divisions of day-to-day labour will in turn produce positive results with respect to health. And while the goal should not be health for the sake of economic productivity it is a fact that better health at the family level will in turn promote economic development as well. Political action groups, men's and women's organisations and youth movements should be seen as appropriate vehicles for community based improvements in maternal and child health.

The coordination between all these sectors, groups and activities should ensure that there is always a well-defined linkeage in their work for, and support of the community. Local committees should be responsible for coordination. A common commitment between sectors to share resources and provide support at all levels is a pre-requisite for the successful grass-roots organization of maternal and child health services.

Regular evaluation and monitoring meetings between community leaders and decision-makers in the various sectors have been shown to be valuable in maintaining the interest of all groups and in ensuring that the community continues to see these administrative networks as legitimate to their needs and expectations.

Meetings of this kind also provide a means by which the different sectors can comment on each others activities and propose improvements. The "competition" potential of such meetings should not be overlooked especially if it can be effectively used for the good of the local community.

16. CONCLUSION - SELF RELIANCE

The message is then that families and communities to achieve appropriate maternal and child health objectives need to be as self reliant as possible. The home provides the essential environment and all services should support it. Central to raising healthy babies is appropriate infant feeding. At the conclusion of the Shanghai Meeting the participants affirmed that there needed to be a target which recognized that most infants in the first few months of their lives should be breastfed. More than this, breastfeeding targets may provide a comprehensive intersectoral purpose that can be the touchstone of development programmes. It may be an indicator as sensitive as infant mortality rates but emphasizing positive signs of self reliant individual and family behaviour, rather than negative results of poverty and inappropriate infant feeding. It is then a social goal par excellence.

It may be true (but more research is needed) that in many poverty situations many mothers breastfeed, but this may simply reflect the inadequacy of standard economic definitions of poverty. Some countries have excellent infant mortality rates without necessarily a high GNP per capita. Certainly countries need to protect breastfeeding as one means of preserving both their independence and the vitality of the coming generation.

The full text of the Shanghai Declaration follows, and it is hoped that it will provide something concrete towards which health and development workers, communities and families can aspire.

THE SHANGHAI DECLARATION
by
THE WHO INTERREGIONAL SEMINAR ON THE ORGANIZATION OF MATERNAL AND CHILD HEALTH SERVICES AT THE GRASS-ROOTS LEVEL

Shanghai - June 1980

1. The basic needs of mothers and children, as defined at the community level are:

- that all pregnancies be healthy and have a safe outcome for both mother and child;
- that there be healthy physical and psychosocial growth and development;
- that there be a safe and healthy environment;
- that children be assured of social, intellectual and emotional stimulation;
- that women have a satisfying social and emotional life.

2. Maternal and child health care must be seen as involving promotive, preventive, curative and rehabilitative care to mothers and children, including family planning.

3. A pre-requisite for effective maternal and child health care is up-dated knowledge about the health states of mothers and children, and regularly collected information that is gathered and used by the community, on the socio-cultural, economic, environmental and health service factors it considers influence health status.

4. The maternal and child health care system must share its knowledge and technology as well as its potentials and limitations with the community, advising and in turn being guided by the community which should be seen as having authority over all services at the grass-roots level.

5. Because most health behaviour is learned at home and because most health care is provided by the family, all social systems and networks both formal and informal, must be oriented to supporting and strengthening this primary unit.

THAT BY 1985 IT BE ENSURED
THAT 80% OR MORE OF ALL INFANTS IN
EVERY COUNTRY BE SOLELY AND ADEQUATELY
BREASTFED FOR AT LEAST FOUR MONTHS

CHAPTER TWO

SELF RELIANT GOALS FOR DEVELOPMENT (1)

1. POVERTY AND DEPRIVATION - A GROWING SPECTRE

There is little doubt that poverty, relative and absolute, is increasing. The least-developed countries are slipping further behind, and increasingly large pockets of poverty are emerging in all countries (the so-called fourth world)(3), especially in rapidly growing, increasingly stratified cities. There are strong suspicions too about the key social indicators (e.g. PQLI (4)) including infant mortality rates and health generally(2). Literacy, too, must surely be affected when it is estimated that 2 out of 3 school-age children in developing countries are not in school but working often in exploitative conditions, even abandoned. Continually and increasingly, people's lives are being disrupted if not destroyed by war, violence and other man-made disasters (9), (10).

2. WHAT'S WRONG WITH EXISTING METHODOLOGIES

The purpose of this paper is to suggest some new methodological approaches, since many present methods seem inadequate. The traditional approach has been to point to a number of quantitative indicators, and to set targets both for the indicators themselves, and for groups on which resources can be concentrated. But, there are very real problems. First, the indicators we have are not always very useful because they may be quite inaccurate. Take infant mortality, for example. There are global estimates from 12 to 50 million p.a. One recent report says that the lack of information is striking (26), and given existing attitudes, organizational infrastructure, etc., this situation is not likely to improve.

As significantly, indicators expressed as national aggregates may obscure internal distributions reflecting very unequal, and probably hardening lines of stratification in power, wealth or status, inequalities which underlie the basic problem of poverty itself.

Indicators, however refined and computerized, tell us very little about the qualitative, especially about what is happening at the grass-roots, and, therefore, little about the great divergence between development objectives, trends and the realities of situations (7).

3. BETTER NUMBER CRUNCHING

A first step is certainly to have new and improved social indicators. For example, UNRISD (6) has put forward very interesting ideas for monitoring at the grass-roots.

There is the new school of rapid (32) research, counting only the essential or highly symbolic (like bars of soap). There has been the suggestion of having an international campaign to count not infant deaths but infant vitality by recording every new birth(5). Hopefully, this would yield data for a more accurate baseline count from which previous indicators could be evaluated retrospectively and more confident future projections made.

4. THE CHILD FOCUS METHODOLOGY

It can be argued, however, that the counting is only the mechanical part and there needs to be other, qualitative methodolgies for integrating socioeconomic approaches. Counting and indicators should not become an end in themselves; it is essential that there is a clear idea of what is being sought. It is important, for instance, in the case of infant vitality, not only to count every new life, but, also, to make every new life count, i.e. to put an emphasis in development objectives on the child. We are suggesting, in fact, a methodology derived from concentrated action for the benefit of particular social groups, rather than abstract econcomic goals (39).

There are a number of reasons for this suggestion in the case of the child. The child has much more political neutrality than many other development objectives and all shades of political opinion are supporting. This was clearly shown during the IYC, and some countries have put the child in the forefront of development objectives (38). Secondly, a concentration of efforts towards the child, is, presumably, an optimal thrust for all the millenial development strategies which promise health or other development benefits by the year 2000, since the children of today are the adults of tomorrow. Thirdly, the problems of the child are closely related to those of women, the two broad groups that have been most abused in the development process. In developing countries there are large number of exploited and abused children(8). Similar methods to those suggested for monitoring and improving the conditions of women could be utilized in child-oriented studies. In fact, it can be argued that the potential of children is not limited to their future involvement in the labour force etc., but they can, themselves, be potent agents of change for other children and even adults in the family or kinship circles (34). Finally, children are central to any "peoples" or intersectoral approaches, and a major focus for self-reliant activities and aspirations.

In many senses, the problems surrounding the child are the problems of development writ small. Gunatilleke (38), for example, in Sri Lanka, has pointed to six deep-seated structural problems which are currently critical to development plans. First, infant mortality rates after an initial drop, and despite increased health services, were only declining slowly. Secondly, nearly 45% of schoolage children did not enter school, or dropped out. Thirdly, and Gunatilleke thought this most important, even those who went to school could not find jobs. Fourthly, there remained groups (e.g. those in the tea plantation areas) who remained much more disadvantaged than others. Fifthly, top-down paternalism, although necessary in the early stages, had gone too far, and urban elites were even directing community development movements. Sixthly, the formal education systems were not encouraging local creativity, based on traditional sources and strengths. This model might well be applied to many developing countries.

To change these situations, to improve the PQLI etc., might not require a vast amount of resources. For example, it has been estimated that infant and child mortality rates could be drastically and dramatically lowered (and, in consequence, life expectancy raised) by a number of quite inexpensive health interventions for the mother and child, for which there is readily available, relatively cheap appropriate technology (24), as well as by improved nutrition which may have longer term effects. Literacy rates might also be improved by some relatively simple health interventions, e.g. the prevention of blindness from vitamin A and D deficiency, or the improvement of deafness by minimizing the effects of upper respiratory infections, or providing low-cost hearing aids. Literacy rate improvements require universal primary schooling, but, if children cannot, or will not go to school, then schools should go out to them, and UNESCO (37), particularly, has recognized the need for reform in this area by a much wider use of informal methods using media which are increasingly available and economic. The ILO has emphasized that employment for all is a feasible objective.

5. THE DEPRIVATION ELEMENT

One point needs special emphasis in all this. Not all children are deprived, and in a world of shrinking resources, there have to be clear priorities, and an awareness of which children need most help.

Basically, the deprived children are the poor children. At first sight the identification of this group seems simple enough. There are those children (some 350 million) who are part of the absolute poor the World Bank has picked out. Some of these children are located in the least-developed countries - perhaps 90 million. But not all poor children are in the LDC's or even amongst those classified amongst the absolute poor. There are estimates as high as 500 million children of school age working or abandoned(30). Not all working children are exploited, but many are, and there is probably a further creation of poverty by the upset caused to the labour market, and increasing unemployment. Then there are the many sick and handicapped and malnourished children under 5, who are such a drain on a poor society, not to mention the time lost to a community which has a high level of infant or child deaths or pregnancies which are not completed for whatever reasons(27). These families are amongst the great majority who are not reached by health and other development services, sometimes in depressed rural areas, in remote mountainous regions and in deserts, but, also, even when they live in urban squatter settlements which are within a stone's throw of urban facilities.

6. TOP DOWN MECHANISMES

Does one, in fact, reach these children by increased resources for health and other development services, through increased political will? Is the answer a welfare-state approach, more health and educational services, etc.? The answer seems to be only partly. The IYC contained many promises, but much less action, and, certainly, the rhetoric needs to be carried forward into resource commitments. Few countries have done this to-date. Certainly, too, as Anell & Nygren (11) have argued, there should be social clauses written into the contracts and relationships which industry (especially the multinationals) and other organizations have with workers and their families. The problems of child labour are undoubtedly(31) created by unregulated industrial activities, just as infant nutrition problems are, in part, explained by inappropriate use of infant food supplements.

But, the redistribution of resources between sectors seems to be only a small part of the answer. There are countries where, for example, health expenditures have risen, but infant mortality rates have remained high(12). Nor is vertical redistribution a complete answer either. The welfare states of developed countries are experiencing extreme problems of costs, and, notably low effectiveness. And the problem is not confined to developed countries. There are examples of food aid which have created more problems than they have solved by creating a dependency or stopping other more vital activities(28). There is some evidence even that introducing money into non-monetized societies may hurt a social fabric based on altruistic dynamics. A story is told in one African village where once everybody took off a day to help build a school or hospital, and brought a brick or a plank. But now there is no building because people expect wages and argue about money anyway. Health and development services have then to be much more sensitive to local structures to be successful, and if they are, a little may go a long way(13).

However, it should be recognized that there are alternative methodologies to the conventional forms of top-down development, whether in a capitalistic or socialistic setting, and even if altered to suit local cultures and conditions. Bottom-up development from below, self-reliance, Sarvodaya, etc. movements have to be examined much more carefully in development plans, and encouraged.

7. A MIDDLE WAY - REINTERPRETING DEVELOPMENT PRIORITIES

This is not, however, a simple argument for bottom-up. The baby should not be thrown out with the bathwater. Some of the early work on the bottom-up approach was rather naive, and did not reflect local realities. Miller (14), for example, has argued for a middle way between top-down and bottom-up. This is a situation where the importance of imported capital and technology declines and locally-generated people-centred ideas increase. All this means some re-thinking of development priorities. First, the idea is not so much basic needs, but rather grass roots aspirations and wants which usually go well beyond basic needs. Secondly, the population/development debate would have to be reviewed and probably turned on its head. In some situations the growth of self reliance would mean an emphasis on labour rather than even the most appropriate non-human capital, and, hence, a tolerance of relatively high population growth rates(35). This would be in tune with many cultures where children and large families are highly valued, where children are regarded even by the well off as a prime investment for the future(36), and where family planning campaigns have often been viewed as an alien intrusion or worse. The results of the latest Indian census just released show how family planning programmes have failed, especially where infant mortality rates remain high. It seems probable that in India at least, and possibly elsewhere, population growth will escalate, and whatever is the theory, this huge reservoir must be used for productive purposes. In situations (particularly in cities), where population growth poses clear problems, the answer may still lie with self reliant institutions by, for example, recognizing and working with the social institutions of the transient squatter settlements and informal economy(15), or finding acceptable ways of accommodating to migration trends.

But, what we need are not theories, but concrete cases. There are, in fact, models which suggest that social development, as expressed, for example, in the PQLI, can be improved in situations of poverty. If, for example, the rankings of PQLI and GNP are compared for countries, there are considerable anomalies. If some countries have wealth without health, others have health without wealth. In fact, even some countries on the UN Least-Developed list figure relatively high on the PQLI ranking(16). More significantly, if one examines differential indicators within countries in different villages, regions, etc., more and more of these anomalies emerge. And the same is true of historical records in many countries.

8. THE SUCCESS STORIES - WHY?

The argument may be put forward that these success stories are very important because they are self-reliant models which should be emulated. A first object of any action research programme should be to identify the causal patterns involved. Our research so far has picked out a number of factors, apart from the importance of child foci. First, there are strong communal organizations. The best may not be those that are purely traditional in character, nor those created by urban elites, but those which blend together local and imported elements. An example in some areas may be cooperative type movements where income generation can be combined with health and educational activities, a mechanism that is showing promise even in urban slum settlements. However, there needs also to be mechanisms for conflict resolution or ensuring the peaceful coexistence of rival ideologies or groups(17), as well as means of reaching individuals and groups at a distance (e.g. the landless), problems which can wreck even the best planned health or development systems(18). There may be excellent health or development services, but, in fact, very few of the countries which have strong PHC movements, for example, have yet achieved startling PQLI; although judgement may be premature since the process is often long and involved(19).

One factor seems common to all success stories: communication. Literacy rates were high, especially female literacy. There were also good communications, not necessarily from the mass media, but, also, in the kinds of integrated, even insular social structure(20) these societies possessed, a structure which favoured a variety of exchanges, including, for example, food and sustenance as well as ideas. All this enabled what butter there was, to be evenly, if thinly, spread in hard times, but also enabled the vital links to the outside to be kept open. Communication was deeply embedded in the culture, and here the traditional milieu was very important.

9. WHAT CAN BE DONE TO HELP?

The first job may, in fact, be to strengthen these communication factors. The means are certainly available to create, at increasingly low cost, a rapid communication system to carry information and knowledge audio-visually to every house in the world. The influence of these media, especially on children and young people, is enormous. On the educational side there is growing experience with open learning systems(21) by which knowledge can be communicated in a flexible and dialogical kind of way(22). All this may be a prime area for international action as commercial interests rapidly monopolize the field. The McBride report, the debate on the new international information order, and its aftermath has highlighted the potentials and the difficulties. But it will be a tragedy if governments are allowed to stop vital information reaching the people themselves.

Of course, it is important that appropriate information is available to all levels of the development system. Here there is certainly a need for new kinds of statistics that are more nearly tailored to the self-reliant issues we have discussed(33). But there is a need for more than this.

In 1980 a very important paper appeared in Human Organization. It was entitled "Toward People's Anthropology", and was written by Fei Xiaotong, in the thirthies, a pioneer applied anthropologist at the London School of Economics, who had gone back to China and had immersed himself for more than 30 years in assisting popular demand, especially of minority groups, for social reform. His people's anthropology is a blend, stressing the scientific collection of data by participant observation, rather than surveys, which becomes the basis not only for making suggestions in the interests of the minority, but helps them also in taking the initiative into their own hands. The paper is critical of some aspects of social development in China when top-down interests muffled these bottom-up dynamics. At the moment there are activities to extend the people's anthropology idea to health and other social development fields(23), and there are many other related and potentially useful action research ideas(25). Such an approach should not only throw light on the basic societal causes of poverty which Jonsson has recently talked about but also provide pragmatic solutions at the local level(40).

The people's anthropology may well provide essential evidence from the complexity of real life situations. This reality may well be put into the communications system, but there remains for there to be effective planning, the need for some translation into a form that is useful to those who plan development. This may be one of the most intriguing challenges of all - how, in short, to marry up the qualitative with the quantitative, putting intellectual and planning ideas at the service of grass-roots movements. This will certainly mean utilizing much more some of the new topological ideas in mathematics (e.g. catastrophe theory) or the synthetic movements in the social sciences (e.g. situational analysis(29), or even creative artists who may well hold the key to stimulating the necessary enthusiasm at the grass-roots in situations where traditional culture is declining.

However, before new methodolgies can be explored and worked out, it can be argued that there is a need for some organizational innovation at the international level. There is probably too much territoriality in the UN system at the moment for any one agency to attack the problem, even if the bureaucratic inertia could be overcome. There is also a need for the inclusion in the process of those outside the intergovernmental structure, e.g. NGO's or industry (here the WHO-UNICEF experience is facilitating the industry - UN-NGO's dialogues might be useful), or the fourth world itself (e.g. drawing on movements such as ATD/Quart Monde, The Fourth World Assembly, etc.). Above all there is a need for a fiercely independent and critical stance, especially on the communications issue, which might involve the new breed of independent NGO's who are emerging or with the traditional repositories of independence - the Universities - who might find for themselves in least-developed, fourth-world, poverty situations a new usefulness and relevance. To help in this process there is a need for specific guidelines and frames to assist workers in the field, as well as concrete goals towards which action-research is pointed(38). Above all, there would need to be a coordinating, animating, facilitating group providing a hothouse for some of these struggling seedlings.

FOOTNOTES

(1) For examples of the literature see Galtung, J.; O'Brien, P.; and, Preiswerk, R. - 1981 - Self Reliance, A Strategy for Development Institute for Development Studies, Geneva. See, also, Footnote 13 below.

(2) Le Monde - 9 September 1981

(3) See the papers from the WHO Fourth World Meeting - Geneva, 19 May 1981. Basically, this meeting saw the fourth world as poor deprived communities, often in cities, not only in the developing countries

(4) See Morris M. Morris - 1979 - Measuring the Conditions of the World's Poor, Oxford, Pergamon. c.f. W. Scott - 1981 - Concepts and Measurements of Poverty - Geneva - UNRISD.

(5) See chapter 12

(6) Scott W. - 1981 - Concepts and Measurement of Poverty, UNRISD - Geneva

(7) UNRISD - 1980 - The Question for a Unified Approach to Development - Geneva

(8) See, e.g. David Pitt and P.M. Shah - 1981 Child Labour and Health in R. Jelliffe (ed.) - Recent Advances in Maternal and Child Health - Oxford University Press, or Defence for Children - 1981 Child Labour - A Threat to the Health and Development - Geneva.

(9) See, e.g. Harfouche, J.K. - 1981 Intra-Species War - A Major Killer of Children in the Third World - What Can We Do About It? in Geneva International Peace Research Institute - 1981 - War and Child Health, Geneva

(10) See R.L. Sivard - 1980 - World Military and Social Expenditure - World Priorities - Virginia, USA. In 1977, US$ 8 per capita was spent on health in the developing world compared with US$ 26 for military purposes. The figure for the developed world was US$ 274 per head for military purposes.

(11) Anell, L. & Nygren, B. 1980 - The Developing Countries and the World Economic Order - London - Methuen

(12) Some middle-eastern countries fall into this category, but it is also true that within countries such as the UK where there is an inverse correlation in some areas between certain kinds of infant mortality and health expenditures and numbers of doctors.

(13) This point was made strongly by E. Schumacher - 1973 - Small is Beautiful - London - Blond & Briggs. c.f. David Pitt - 1976 - The Social Dynamics of Development Oxford and (ed) Development From Below (Mouton)

(14) Miller, E. - 1974 - The Negotiating Model in W.C. Lawrence (ed) - Exploring Individual and Organizational Boundaries - London - Wiley

(15) c.f. K. Yusof's chapter in this book. IKETSETSENG Paper, WHO/MCH, Geneva

(16) The best examples are in Samoa, but many low income countries (Sri Lanka, Caribbean Islands) or districts (Kerala, India) score well.

(17) For an example, David Pitt - 1970 - Tradition and Economic Progress - Oxford University Press

(18) For an example of such a wrecked scheme, see Williams, G. & Satato's Indonesian evidence in Development Dialogue, 1980, 2.1

(19) See, e.g. WHO/UNICEF JCHP Study - 1981 - National Decision Making for Primary Health Care, Geneva

(20) On the relationships of Islands to Development, see Edouard Dommen (ed) - 1981 - Islands and Development - Oxford - Pergamon

(21) See David Pitt - 1981 - Open House - WHO/MCH, Geneva unpublished paper.

(22) c.f. David Werner - 1981 - Where there is no Doctor - London, MacMillan

(23) E.g. David Pitt - 1981 - The People's Anthropology and Child Health - WHO/MCH, Geneva, unpublished paper.

(24) E.g. Immunization could eradicate neonatal tetanus and reduce many childhood diseases: diphtheria, measles, polio, etc. See WHO - 1980 - Towards a Better Future Geneva, p. 34 ff.

(25) See, e.g. The International Journal of Community Development, 1980, No. 2

(26) D. McGranahan - 1980 - Improvement of Information on the Condition of Children, UNRISD, Geneva

(27) See, for example, Solomon Ayalew - in chapter 9

(28) See Chapter 4

(29) See, e.g. Magnusson, D. & Endler, N. - 1977 - Personality at the Crossroads - Erlbaum, J.G., for a popular account- see Michael Argyle - 1981 - The Situational Approach to Social Problems - New Society, 14 May 1981

(30) Not all these children are sick, and some may be part of self-sufficient gangs, etc., which may have potential even if they are presently usually on the wrong side of the law. But it has been estimated that 10% of children in developing countries are handicapped, and most of the latter-day Robin Hoods live in most unsanitary and unhealthy conditions. On the handicapped, see - Moyes, A - 1981 - One in 10 - Oxfam.

(31) See, e.g. Adelwahab Bouhdiba - Exploitation of Child Labour - UNECOSOC/Doc. E/CN.4/Sub.2/479, p.45 ff

(32) See Pacey, M - Taking Soundings in Developing Countries - WHO/FHE, Geneva - 1981

(33) E.g. I. Palmer & U. von Buchwald - 1980 - Monitoring Changes in the Conditions of Women - UNRISD - Geneva

(34) A good example is the child-to-child programme at the University of London

(35) c.f. Ester Boserups enlargement of her thesis that population changes are crucial to economic development rather than vice-versa. 1981 - Population and Technological Change - A Study of Long-Term Trends - University of Chicago Press

(36) See Asok Mitra - A commentary on the Indian Census - The Statesman - New Delhi - 5 October 1981

(37) See, e.g. UNESCO - 1980 - Consultation interagence sur les besoins de l'enfant - Document de travail principal - ED/SCM/CUR/AIE/435

(38) See, for example, Gunatilleke, G. 1 - 1981 - Changing Needs of Children - The Experience of Sri Lanka - Marga Institute - Colombo. Gunatilleke has identified 3 concrete goals as a major part of a development strategy, a reduction in infant mortality rates to 2.5%, the elimination of malnutrition, universal primary education for the 5-9 years age group.

(39) For a clear statement, see Sterky, G., Nordberg, O. & Philipps, P. - 1975 - Action for Children - Uppsala - Dag Hammarskjold Foundation

(40) U. Jonsson - 1981 - The Causes of Hunger - UNU - Food & Nutrition Bulletin V.3.10.2

CHAPTER THREE

HEALTH WITHOUT WEALTH

1. HEALTH AND DEVELOPMENT - TOO MUCH THEORY

In the recent discussions on health and development(1), there has been much confusion about relationships and causes, a confusion which has not helped those working in developing countries. Some have avoided the issue by making both health and development the same, under the umbrella of well being. For others, health is either, or sometimes both, the cause or effect of development regarded as economic growth. The assumption is that the attack on poverty, by fulfilling basic needs, will result in both better health and development. Much of the confusion has come from the theoretical nature of the argument far removed from the realities of the field. Portmanteau concepts like health/development, even primary health care, communities, peasants, etc. are not very useful unless applied to specific situations. What this brief paper tries to do is to pick on some interesting and sometimes neglected specific situations to try to show more precisely what the relationship is between health and development, and how this might be used in plans for health and development for all by the year 2000.

2. MEASURING HEALTH AND DEVELOPMENT - SOME IMPERFECT INDICATORS

First, we need to have some way of evaluating what a succesful health/development situation is. There are several fashionable ways of measuring either or both at the moment. Most popular is PQLI(2) - the Physical Quality of Life Index (or its historical application - Disparity Reduction Rates). PQLI combines infant mortality rates (IMR), expectation of life and literacy. Others, including the opponents of PQLI, have used IMR or expectation of life as single indicators, or have moved to more innovative ideas such as Low Birthweight (3). Wealth has been measured particularly by Gross National Product (GNP per capita)(5).

There are all sorts of problems with these indicators. The key indicator, IMR, is often wildly exaggerated in official reports, or vastly underreported because of inadequate registration procedures, whilst indirect estimation is also tricky because of census irregularities. Too seldom IMR has been linked with child mortality or morbidity rates, which may increase if IMR goes down. The weighting of PQLI is inevitably arbitrary. GNP has been widely and probably justly criticized. GNP does not include subsistence, does not measure the internal distribution of wealth, especially those living below a minimum wealth level. GNP may only reflect fluctuating exchange rates. There is a desperate need for new and improved indicators on which to base planning and a simple means whereby communities can collect their own data and even formulate their own indicators.

A second, major problem is that statistics aggregate in space and time. In reality, every country is a constantly changing mixture of succesful and failing regions, communities and social groups (4).

3. SUCCESS STORIES

Absolute we cannot be, but nonetheless, it is possible to produce names of countries (26) and regions which have done relatively well in health without much wealth, and whose example might well be useful to others. There are groups of countries, for instance, which have relatively low IMRs (probably below 40 o/oo), good PQLIs and a GNP per capita below $700(5). Then there are situations where GNP per capita is higher, say, up to around $2,000 per annum per capita, and where the IMR probably drops below 30 o/oo(36). Then there are those countries with high disparity reduction rates (i.e. basically rapidly improving PQLI(37). Finally, using World Bank indicators of wealth and expectation of life, there is yet another list of successful paradigms(35).

There are all sorts of problems with these lists. We simply do not often know the relative reliability of statistics, especially when official and other estimates vary. There is little in them to measure the success of particular villages (notably in Africa)(9), or future potential, which is considerable in some countries(10). Much of the material is at least 5 years out of date, and may be quite irrelevant in those countries which have experienced recent dramatic changes (e.g. energy crisis, wars, revolutions, etc.). Bear in mind, then, that our lists are partial.

4. WHAT ARE NOT EXPLANATIONS

One thing is immediately interesting about all these lists. There is a range of social, economic and political systems, cultures, regions, colonial histories and so on. All of which is reflected in the range of health care systems(39). But there are some features which most countries on the list did not have. These were not(23) countries, for example, with huge foreign aid, exceptional natural resources or advantageous terms of trade. Stewart(33) remarked that although many developed countries espoused the cause of basic needs, there has been little support for those countries which have tried to meet basic needs and even (in the case of Sri Lanka) attempts at dismantling the system so that direct foreign exchange costs of projects could be financed. The answer then was not aid or trade.

5. HEALTH SERVICES - QUALITY NOT QUANTITY, AND, ONLY THEN PART OF THE STORY

One certain factor in the explanation of succes is that in policy and planning a prominent place is given to social as opposed to economic development, and to providing for basic needs, including Primary Health Care. There is, to use the cliché, a political will to improve health, not so much through expensive curative services, but through prevention and a comprehensive public health system which reaches rural and slum areas. This may be measured by money spent in budgets on health, or numbers of health personnel, or hospital beds. Quantity and quality are, however, not necessarily related(15), and there have been those who have pointed to the so called "doctor" anomaly(6) where there is a negative correlation in terms of IMR. This may be a chicken and egg kind of problem, health resources being attracted to poor areas(17), or the results, as Chalmers and others have argued, of inappropriate technology(18). Certainly, there are some countries where there is a clear result from large expenditure. Cuba, for example, has spent about twice as much of its national income on health education as other developing countries with a similar income level. There are clearly alternative roads, and it has been argued(35) that one is where government investment goes into creating a labour-intensive economy with employment opportunities. Families receive, therefore, higher incomes which they can use for meeting basic needs, buying better food, etc. The Republic of Korea and Taiwan are good examples of this process.

The countries we are talking about are, in fact, at varying points on the scale of health expenditure however calculated(7). More important may be the degree to which intersectoral action allows resources to be used effectively to the extent to which the health services are "barefoot", i.e. in real contact and communication with the communities on the periphery of the social structure, in the countryside and slums, away from the wealthier urban areas.

And, most important in all cases, MCH has a prominent place in the health services pattern. The longer the time MCH is a central feature of government policies, the better the effects. In Sri Lanka the MCH emphasis appeared in the nineteen-thirties. This emphasis needs to be more than an phrase tripped off the tongue during the International Year of the Child, or relegated to the female power structure surrounding the "first lady". It should be written concretely into national development plans. As Patel has shown in Sri Lanka(8), this was not a question of a simple relationship with money spent, for as the MCH budget went up, IMR stayed constant.

MCH is often linked with family planning, and certainly, in some of the countries we are talking about population increase rates are relatively low, and the rates of women using contraception relatively high(24). But there were exceptions (e.g. W.Samoa). In some cases, too, improvement in IMR came before declines in population, probably reflecting the importance of IM in people's reasons for having large families. The population issue may, in fact, be something of a red herring. Nag has shown how(27) high fertility and high income can be related, and the same may be true of low fertility and low income.

6. PRIMARY HEALTH CARE (PHC) - A PIOUS BUT EXPENSIVE HOPE

MCH is a fundamental part of PHC, but there can be less certainty about the other parts of the PHC package that was produced at the 1978 WHO/UNICEF Conference in Alma-Ata. PHC is a new idea, even if something of a transmogrified basic services, and it is clearly too early to tell in many areas. PHC has elements still of top-down, even if expressed in botton-up language. Worse still, it looks very expensive. Recent estimates(7) have pointed to a figure of 103 billion US$ (1978 rates) to finance PHC by the year 2000. Developing countries would have to pay, in some cases, 10 times what they are now paying, whilst outside aid would have to triple. Put simply, few countries may buy it.

There may be ways round the problem, e.g. concentrating on certain diseases, but it might be asked whether the game is worth the candle. For example, there is evidence from Sri Lanka(8) of a wide variation in the correlation in different districts of water sanitation and IMR and the countries we are talking about generally do not have excellent water indicators(25). Essential drugs are not readily available, nor is there necessarily good health education.

Improving overall levels of nutrition is only part of the story, too. The Kerala information(28) here is fascinating. A number of studies have shown that food intake in Kerala is low, lower than a number of other Indian states, yet infant mortality rates are the lowest, (especially female infant mortality rates) by some way of all Indian States. There is also a longer expectation of life. The United Nations study of Kerala argued that other factors were as important, perhaps more important than nutrition, particularly medical (including ayurvedic) services where the utilization rate was also the highest in India. Although expenditure was not the highest, it was more equitably distributed. There is little doubt that health services made a contribution, but it was probably not the critical causal agent. The point about distribution is probably more important, since it enabled relatively less food to be spread more thinly and effectively.

The essential seems to be that PHC cannot work unless and until there is an appropriate social environment which allows the elements of PHC to be shared by a wide range of people. This means not only, or not mainly, government prerogatives, but, also, popular will, strong community structures and mechanisms to promote development from below(13).

7. CERTAIN KINDS OF SOCIAL STRUCTURES

What sort of social structure did these success stories have? One superficial observation is that there are a large number of islands in the group. Some recent studies(11) have shown how islands favour strong social pressures and good communications. But islands also feature amongst some of the failures, and it may be that islands are more exposed to periodic disasters (e.g. epidemic as opposed to endemic disease, climatic disasters, etc.).

There are clearly other factors at work. One is certainly strong community structures. This was also a reason why promising, outside institutions were able to be absorbed. For example, Jamaica, Trinidad, Mauritius, Sri Lanka have all strong cooperative movements. In Sri Lanka these are 7,500 with a membership of 1.8 million concerned with credit, distribution of consumer goods and production. Special attention is given to cooperatives in rural development under the Land Reform Act. Chinese communes are another example of a development from cooperatives(12).

As important is the absence of rigid social stratification, and the presence of social mobility, features found in both capitalist(14) and socialist situations. Studies(26) of IMR rates in Cuba show how improvements can come before the political revolution. The redistribution of wealth was particularly important. It needed to flow, not trickle down, and all the countries showed recent important improvements in the proportions of wealth held by low-income families.

It was especially important that food should be redistributed equitably. In rural areas this implied access to subsistence(29) land and/or the cash rewards for working the land. Most of the countries we are talking about had land reform schemes, and reasonably high indices of food production(22) Significantly, the levels of the poorest household were being raised at relatively fast rates(34). In Sri Lanka this was due to government intervention, where, for example, the food ration scheme from 1973 amounted to 14% of the income of the poorest families (or 20% of calorie intake). Significantly, too, inflation rates were not great(21). In many respects, there was a balance between labour and capital, and certainly not the labour-intensive situation which produced the vicious circle of agricultural involution that Clifford Geertz has described(20).

Part of the reason for redistribution was the relatively good lines of communication, especially between urban and rurual areas, along which there could be a flow of information and capital. Not all this communication was in western forms, though education, literacy and, in some cases mass media, were all well developed. There were some traditional methods, e.g. the Malaga walking party in Samoa, or posters and loudspeakers in China. Of course, in the stratification system there were conflicting interests and pressures. But there also seemed to be mechanisms to resolve them. For example, Williams and Satoto(19) have recently described in Indonesia how conflict in a village prevented the full realization of PHC, basically because the existing authorities in the village did not want a rival power structure. By contrast, many of the villages we are talking about were able to accommodate to this situation of conflict either because the "traditional" authorities were flexible enough to add a new function to their bag, or because there existed in the village a pluralistic structure which allowed two or more power streams to coexist(29).

The real significance of the Indonesian example was that the conflict effectively killed the fragile flower of motivation amongst the people, e.g. mothers no longer came to the clinics. In the success stories by contrast, this motivation was positively cumulative, once set off it multiplied and spread to other sectors.

Although there has been considerable literature on the effects of stratification in space, there has been much less attention paid to the time dimension which may be as important. People may be poor at one time, and not another, and often there is a succession of lean and fat years. Chambers(31) has recently shown how seasons are critical to the health of the landless and the poor. The times or risk and danger, rather than social group risk factors is one of the most important, neglected areas for health interventions. As Gibb(32) argued, it is the way in which the social organization copes with these rhythms that is critical. Too often there is not adequate planning which would allow a continuous supply of vital foods or essential drugs, etc.

8. THE STATUS OF WOMEN - A MUST

One essential corollary of health without wealth seems to be the status of women. In all the countries we are talking about, female literacy was relatively high. As Caldwell(14) and others have argued, this was not just a reflection of improved standards of living, but a more fundamental social change.

The more educated the woman is, the more knowledge she will have to help her in her pregnancy. She will be more able to manipulate the outside world, feel personal responsibility and challenge outmoded and inappropriate authorities (e.g. many mothers-in-law) and to communicate with her husband. She is more likely to be child-centred and to lavish more attention on her child. This is no small factor, for maternal neglect has been cited as a major reason for the high rates of female infant mortality that are found in parts of India. It is interesting that Kerala has the lowest female infant mortality rates of all the Indian States and a relationship of male-to-female IMRs similar to industrialized countries.

The status of women is reflected in the ways in which the critical period of birth is handled itself. Sri Lanka seems to be a case where a major improvement in IMR was achieved by mothers stopping unfortunate traditional practices, e.g. using dung as a healing agent after the severing of the umbilical cord which led to fatal tetanus neonatorum, or the habit of giving an infant only castor oil and sugar for three days, so upsetting both the infants digestive system and the mother's lactational cycle(8). The point here is not that traditional practices are necessarily bad; there are other reports (e.g. from Samoa) of traditional pregnancy taboos that were beneficial, but rather that the mother could make an informed choice. The level of female education was important too in the quality of the birth attendants whose intervention was most significant, especially when there were complications.

9. THE STATUS OF THE CHILD - ANOTHER MUST

As important as the status of women is the status of the child, and the two are both necessary(38). As a rough rule of thumb it seems that where children are highly valued, IMR rates are lowest. One reason that has been put forward for the very high rates of IMR in parts of early, modern Europe (much higher than most developing countries today incidentally) has been the fact that children were not regarded fully as people. They were given away to wet nurses who, once they received their payment, no longer cared for them. Parents sometimes did not know how many children they had, and never even went to their funerals(16). They were used and abused as child labour. The countries we are talking about seem much more child centred. In some cases, this value was expressed through having a large, extended family network (e.g. Samoa), in other cases through a nuclear family emphasis, often with a relatively late marriage pattern. Here, the small numbers of children made it imperative that the best pre- and post-natal care was sought. Exploitative child labour was not common. School numbers were higher. The numbers of abandoned children were much less than elsewhere. The sick child seems to have been relatively well cared for in the home, and neither neglected nor incarcerated for long periods in hospitals remote from their loved ones. The sick child was not then treated as an outcast or deviant.

10. SOME CONCLUDING QUESTIONS

In summary, it seems as if it would be a good idea if those who plan and implement social development could ask themselves and the communities some searching questions:

i) is it possible to achieve health and wellbeing without a large, expensive bureaucracy? This is a question of great relevance to welfare states in developed countries too;

ii) what mechanisms are needed at the community level to accomplish health/development from below? How relevant are the experiences of the "Health Without Wealth" countries and communities?

iii) what are the sectors (education? agriculture?) etc. whose support would best further health and development?;

iv) what can be done immediately to improve the lot of women and children, and to improve their opportunities in life? What are the critical interventions, the ways of breaking the vicious circles(30) that are the curse of the third world?

FOOTNOTES

(1) See Grosse R. N. and Harkavy O - 1980- The Role of Health in Development - Social Science and Medicine, Vol. 14C, p.165-167, or McEvers N.C. - 1980 - Health and the Assault on Poverty in Low-Income Countries - Social Science and Medicine, Vol. 14C, p.41-57. (especially the latter) has a good bibliography.

(2) See Morris D. Morris - 1979 - Measuring the Condition of the World's Poor - Oxford-Pergamon; Grant J. - 1978 - Disparity Reduction Rates - ODI - Washington. A critique of PQLI is in Streeten P. and Hicks in Development Digest 1980. On IMR, cf Vallin J. - 1976 - World Trends in IMR Since 1950 - World Statistics Report 29-646-74.

(3) e.g. Sterky G. and Mellander L. (eds.) - 1978 - Birthweight Distribution - An Indicator of Social Development - SAREC - Uppsala.

(4) cf Fei Xiaotong - 1980 - Towards a People's Anthropology - Applied Anthropology, Vol. 39, No. 2. The studies of Redfield and Oscar Lewis in a village Tepotzlan, Mexico, probably shows how social structures may change quite rapidly.

(5) PQLI and GNP figures are from Morris op.cit. 1979, whilst Infant Mortality Rates are from the Population Reference Bureau, Washington (1980) - World's Children Data Sheet. The list is Cuba, Western Samoa, Sri Lanka, Mauritius, parts of China, Kerala (India).

(6) e.g. Cochrane A. et al. - 1978 - Health Service Input and Mortality Output - Journal of Epidemiology and Community Health, Vol. 32, p.200-205.

(7) See Joseph S.C. and Russel S.S. - 1980 - Is Primary Care the Wave of the Future? - Social Science and Medicine, Vol. 14C, p.137-144. Figures on numbers of health personnel are in World Development Report - August, 1980 - Taking 3 of our countries for example: in Sri Lanka the per capita public health expenditure was 2.3% of GNP per capita; in China it was 1.0%; and in the Republic of Korea, 0.3% compared to countries such as Papua-New Guinea, Ivory Coast, etc. where the figure was over 5%.

(8) Patel M. - 1980 - Effects of Health Service and Environmental Factors on Infant Mortality - The Case of Sri Lanka - Journal of Epidemiology and Community Health, Vol. 34, No.-2, p.76-82.

(9) cf Wenlock R. - 1979 - Social Factors, Nutrition and Child Mortality in a Rural Subsistence Economy - Ecology of Food and Nutrition 8, 227-240

(10) e.g. Mozambique and Tanzania - cf Moore F.L. and Becla A. - Kerala - Asking the Big Questions - San Francisco - Institute for Food and Development Policy.

(11) On the theme of Islands and Development, see the special issue of World Development, No.1, 1981, especially the chapters by Edward Dommen and David Pitt.

(12) There is a good pupular account in Harrison Paul - 1980 - The Third World Tomorrow - London-Penguin.

(13) For examples, see Pitt D. - 1976 - Social Dynamics of Development - Oxford-Pergamon and (Ed) Development From Below - Paris and the Hague-Mouton. A case study of Samoa is Pitt D. - 1970 - Tradition and Economic Progress - Oxford University Press.

(14) Caldwell J.C. - 1979 - Education as a Factor in Mortality Decline - Population Studies, Vol. 33, p.395-413.

(15) cf McKeown T. - 1976 - The Modern Rise of Population - London-Arnold

(16) See Burke P. In Doxiadis B. - (Ed) - 1979 - The Child in the World of Tomorrow - Oxford-Pergamon.

(17) For an interesting theory on sickness as a crime, see Dubos R. - 1959 - The Mirage of Health - New York-Harper.

(18) cf Chalmers I. and Richards M.P.N. - 1977 - Benefits and Hazards of the New Obstetrics - Ed. Charde T. and Richards - London-Heinemann.

(19) Williams G. and Satoto - 1980 - Socio-Political Constraints on PHC - Development Dialogue, Vol. 1, p.85-102.

(20) Geertz C. - 1968 - Agricultural Involution - University of California Press.

(21) Though, Trinidad, Jamaica, Republic of Korea all had an inflation rate of over 15% for the years 1976-1978 - World Bank 1980, World Development Report, p.110.

(22) In 1976-1978 - e.g. Sri Lanka had an index of 116 compared to the the Low-Income Country average of 97 - World Bank 1980, World Development Report 1980, p.110.

(23) cf World Bank 1980 - World Development Report Tables, p.110.

(24) In no case (apart from Samoa) was the annual growth rate (1970-1978) over 2.0%. The percentage of married women using contraceptives was relatively high in, for example, Sri Lanka in 1977 (41%) though not in 1970 (8%). It was even high in Taiwan in both years (44%, 65%). World Bank 1980, World Development Report. Tables 17, 18.

(25) Sri Lanka, e.g. had only 20% of the population in 1975 with access to safe water, well below the low income country average according to the World Bank. Cf. a later "rapid" assessment by World Bank who gave 45% (urban) and 13% (rural) with the corresponding figures for adequate sanitation 80% and 56%. The safe water figure for Samoa was 23%. World Bank 1980 - World Development Report, Table 22.

(26) Some selected sources on the situations listed below are in China - David Milton et al - 1977 - People's China - Penguin; Cuba - UNCTAD - 1979 - Health and Educational Technology in Cuba - Geneva; and Roemer M. - 1976 - Cuban Health Services - Washington-PAHO; Sri Lanka - Marga Quarterly - 1978 - Participatory Development and Dependence - Vol. 5, No. 3; and Simeonoul - 1975 - Better Health for Sri Lanka - WHO, SEARO.

(27) In Current Anthropology - October 1980.

(28) Centre for Developing Studies - 1975 - India, Poverty, Unemployment and Development Policy - United Nations, New York.

(29) See Pitt D. - 1970 - Tradition and Economic Progress - Oxford University Press.

(30) Elmendorf Mary - 1980 - Women, Water and Waste - Equity Policy Centre, Washington has argued that a simple way of breaking the oral-faecial infection cycle is to have several buckets that are covered and used only for one purpose.

(31) Chambers R. - 1979 - Health, Agriculture and Rural Poverty - Why Seasons Matter - Discussion Paper 148, IDS-Sussex.

(32) World Meteorological Organization Paper presented to the UN Meeting on Population, Resources, Environment and Development - Geneva, July 1980.

(33) Stewart F. - 1979 - The NIEO and Basic Needs - Nordic Symposium on Development Strategies, Research Policy Institute, University of Lund, Sweden.

(34) Stewart op.cit. Selowsky M. - 1979 - Balancing Trickle Down and Basic Needs - Strategies - World Bank, Washington. In Sri Lanka, for example, the lowest household decile increased its share of income by 105% in the years 1963-1973 whilst the top decile reduced by 17.2%. Marga Institute op.cit.

(35) See Frances Stewart - 1979 - Country Experience in Providing for Basic Needs - Finance and Development, Vol. 16.

(36) Included would be Singapore, Hong Kong, Malta, Jamaica, Bulgaria, Taiwan, Cyprus, Barbados.

(37) Those countries with over 3% p.a. DRR are Mauritius, Korea (Republic of), Yugoslavia, Jamaica, Cyprus, Trinidad, Costa Rica, Hong Kong, Taiwan.

(38) c.f. Maya Chadola - 1980 - Women but not children first - Populi, Vol. 7, No.2, p.24-32.

(39) Milton Roemer - 1977 - Comparative National Policies on Health Care - New York - Dekker has isolated five main types of health care system - free enterprise, welfare state, underdeveloped, transitional socialist.

CHAPTER FOUR

DISHING OUT - ALTERNATIVE SELF RELIANT MEANS FOR FEEDING MOTHERS AND CHILDREN

1. LOGIC OF FOOD AID

It is usually thought that the problems of poverty are closely related to problems of hunger. To improve maternal and child health it is simply necessary to feed mothers and children better. To take the food from those countries with a food surplus and to redistribute it to the poor nations. To most development problems, simple answers are given, but the most simple answers are often wrong, or, at least, not completely right. Of course, improved nutrition is vital to maternal and child health, but we are dealing with different, separate systems, and in some situations, they may work against each other. In this brief paper we examine the particular case of the distribution of food aid through health installations.

Food aid is given for all kinds or purposes in the Third World. It is used to relieve emergency situations such as wars and similar disasters. It is given to refugees. It is used as an incentive to encourage people to use various government services, whilst, at the same time, providing them with much-needed nutrition. It is this last problem that we are concerned with here.

The logic of food aid schemes is obvious enough. The average level of nutrition in a country may be low, but this is not to say that those who need the food most will get it, or that it will solve their nutrition or health problems in the long term. What follows is not meant to be a negative criticism of all food aid. In disaster situations there has to be food aid. In many ordinary situations too it works well(2) but reports from the grass-roots suggest there are serious unintended, often unrecognized problems, for which constructive solutions need to be found(1).

2. ADVERSE EFFECT IN GENERAL

Food aid may create several kinds of adverse effects. Somebody has said that aid is the money given by the poor people in rich countries to the rich people in poor countries. Food may go to people who do not need it, who may sell it, give it to animals, let it rot, etc. Inevitably, black markets develop. When there is a surfeit of food, there is a greater tendency to wastage, and ineffective distribution. Corruption is common.

Often food aid destroys self reliance, and creates dependancy on foods imported from outside the country. The distribution of infant foods may disrupt beneficial traditional practices, such as breastfeeding. When food is cooked it tends to undermine the continuation of valuable culinary skills. When the aid dries up, imported foods can be an unbearable strain on foreign exchange resources. Sometimes the food imported is culturally inappropriate so that it is rejected by the people or fed to animals.

Most of these facts are well known and well documented. The effects on maternal and child health are indirect, if still considerable.

3. ADVERSE EFFECTS ON MATERNAL AND CHILD HEALTH

Less well known are the ways in which a food distribution system can restrict or even destroy a primary health care system, and, in particular, its maternal and child health functions.

A typical situation in many countries may develop in the following fashion:
The staff in Maternal and Child Health clinics have to work hard to build up their services, and often the hardest work is to establish credibility and acceptability in the eyes of the local population. Maternal and child health services are frequently understood to consist of routine procedures, e.g. weighing the mother and baby, injecting the baby which makes him or her cry, and may even give him or her a fever. None of these procedures are seen by the local people to have immediate benefits. The mother and baby may have to walk many hours, and, in some countries, days to reach the clinic and wait a long time in unfamiliar and sometimes unfriendly situations. Then there is suddenly "Food Aid" operating, and news reaches the local population that by going to the clinic you may be able to obtain, free of charge, let us say, a bottle of oil, 2 1/2 kg of bulgar wheat, 4 kg of blended flour, whereupon the long journey to the clinic appears more worthwhile. The news of this new benefit spreads very fast, and, rather quickly, more and more mothers are making the journey to the clinic. The clinic staff suddenly

have to provide services to greatly increased numbers. This sudden, rapidly increased work-load creates a problem in itself - the staff do their best to abide by the planned order of work which may be roughly as follows:

- Provide routine antenatal care to the mother;
- examine the child/children with her;
- give appropriate counselling and/or treatment;
- give any immunizations which are due;
- organize and give group health education session(s)

after which comes the long-awaited food "hand-out". As the day wears on and many mothers are still waiting to be seen, and they have a long way to go to return home, the staff of the clinic, not wishing to send anyone away dissatisfied, and knowing that the priority in the minds of the mothers is the food, are tempted to give them the food and let them return home, satisfied, but unseen. They rationalize the position by saying that the examinations, etc. can be done at the next visit. Thus, a self-perpetuating situation can arise in which the handing-out of food takes precedence over other tasks such as examining mothers and babies, counselling, etc., and, worst of all over even the immunizations. The final "insult" comes when, having "adjusted" the work of the clinic to this situation, there may come a time when the food supplies are temporarily or permanently stopped and thereupon the clinic also "stops" since many mothers may not then bother to come any more to this clinic or other facilities.

At best there is a loss of morale amongst staff and an unfortunate expectation amongst mothers. The strength of this expectation makes it difficult to switch into other courses of action, for example, giving the mothers seeds and asking them to plant them and grow their own food.

In any case, this is usually very difficult since food donor agencies are reluctant to abandon their accepted role and to move into a new, often jealously guarded activity (in this case, agriculture) whilst there is often a local resistance to outsiders telling them how to grow local foods which they have done for years. Governments, fearing political repercussions, try to keep the ragged populace happy with bread, if not circuses.

But, worse than being locked into a food distribution role is the degeneration of the programme into mendacity. In one country where the respectable women of the community could not, by local mores, come out of their homes, the clinics became centres for food collection by beggars and had to be closed because of the protests of the elders of the community.

4. SOLUTIONS - FROM ABOVE

Such is the problem. What are the solutions? First, there is the solution "from above", because like many development problems, the failure of food aid is the failure of effective management. There is too little coordination amongst the agencies, and with the various government departments, there is too little rational planning of distribution in space and time. There is too little information or identification of those groups who are most in need. There is inadequate planning of strategies to screen and reach those groups in need. There is too little consultation with local communities themselves.

5. SOLUTIONS - THE NEED FOR SELF RELIANCE

However, even if the big management problems are solved, there remains the problem that the general relationship between food aid and maternal and child health is unsatisfactory, and, more significantly, that much more needs to be done to strengthen local organizations. There needs to be an institutional self reliance which might ultimately spread into agriculture and food production. To some degree, disaster situations are excepted from this, but even here the value of self reliance should not be underestimated.

In this process, of course, the maternal and child health facilities can play an important role. In fact, with the clinics must rest the essential task of screening out those mothers and babies that do need the nutritional supplements. But the task of feeding should be carried out elsewhere. Exactly where may vary from country to country, or community to community, since each will have its own strong and weak points.

6. SOLUTIONS - FROM LESOTHO

As an example, a range of alternative solutions have been suggested from Lesotho. The country has a very difficult terrain, poor communications and problems of manpower, not least because many men (and women health workers) have migrated to South Africa. Indeed, much of Lesotho's wealth is derived from migrant remittances. There is an extensive food aid programme distributed by the World Food Programme and Catholic Relief Services donated particularly by the USA. Many of Lesotho's 85 clinics provide food aid (90% of people going to them receive food for their children). The dishing-out syndrome we have described is found in some of the Lesotho clinics. The average travel time to a clinic for mothers is three hours. Malnutrition (PEM) is probably not high but infant mortality rates are estimated to be 11.4%. Critics of the school feeding programme have also claimed that the target groups are not being reached and there have been claims that only the pigs are getting fat.

The following solutions have been suggested by the local health workers. After simple screening procedures by health workers, the undernourished should be referred to one or more of the following:

- group feeding centres which can be implemented at community level rather than being solely dependent upon health facilities;
- women's organizations, which might be motivated to voluntarily execute feeding programmes for those at risk at various points throughout the country, using schools, churches, court rooms, and other prominent places where people easily gather;
- cooperatives; donated food could be sold at reduced prices, and the money used for other development activities in the community when food is not actually needed;
- food canteens; where food is sold at reduced prices for those at work, those in the low income groups and those with large families;
- social centres, clubs, nutrition centres, nutrition rehabilitation centres;
- food stores, built at different points and filled with emergency food commodities for relief during emergencies (e.g. the present drought);
- food stamps or ration coupons which could be issued for those in need.

7. POSSIBILITIES - SEVERAL FRONTS

The Lesotho suggestions are very interesting. They show clearly that it is necessary to approach the problem on a number of fronts. Not all institutions will or can work, and a certain amount of experiment and much dialogue is needed to find the most effective solution, about which there is the greatest consensus.

8. POSSIBILITIES - COOPERATIVES

Secondly, there is the possibility which exists in many countries of revitalizing the cooperative movement. Cooperatives have had many critics and many failures, but they still can provide a middle way between the excessive individualism of laissez-faire capitalism and the overbearing imposition of centralized state institutions. In a world still based on market forces, cooperatives remain a means of collectively cushioning members from the threats of overwhelming costs and prices. There are important spin-offs too especially in education, and cooperatives have shown in many countries that there are possibilities of providing a wide range of social services.

9. POSSIBILITIES - WOMEN'S GROUPS

Possibly the most interesting feature of the Lesotho situation is the prime role that women have played and might play. Women, and especially mothers, have been a neglected positive force in the third world, and the vital problem of mother and child feeding is an area in which their many talents might be amply demonstrated.

10. POSSIBILITIES - BOLIVIAN MOTHER'S CLUBS

Lesotho is not the only country which is thinking of using mothers' organizations in achieving maternal and child health objectives through improved feeding schemes. In Bolivia, for example, since 1972 the mothers' clubs (created under the Ministry of Health and Social Welfare), in rural and marginal urban areas, have provided the organizational structure for these activities. This programme has a staff of nutritionists, auxiliary nutritionists, nurses, auxiliary nurses and social workers, for the technical aspects of the programme and for the distribution of food.

The Nutrition Division assists some 600 mothers' clubs, and through them, provides the following five main programmes:

a) Social promotion activities;

b) preventive medicine;

c) vaccinations;

d) control of child growth;

e) food assistance.

Within these programmes, special attention is given to nutrition and health education. Mothers pay a small membership fee and have the right to food rations after attending four consecutive meetings.

The mothers' clubs are at different stages of development with regard to their cohesion as groups, ability in contributing to the achievement of the objectives of the programme, in taking initiatives to expand their activities, and to solve some of their own problems. Some of the mothers' clubs with four to five years of experience have been able to accumulate funds in amounts varying from club to club and according to size of membership. The funds have been invested in various productive activities.

The management skill of each club is reflected in the type of activities undertaken, amount of profit, recovery of the funds and future plans for investment. Some clubs buy food, household articles, school materials, equipment and materials for handicrafts or other small industries, clothing, etc., to be sold to their members at prices lower than those prevailing in the market. Others have undertaken some community projects, such as drinking water facilities for the homes, construction of latrines and social activities. These activities are developed under the supervision of the nutrition staff and constitute the initial stage of a pre-cooperative system. Through this team work the clubs have gained experience which provides them with a sound basis to develop later a cooperative system.

With the continuation and strengthening of this programme, the Government intends not only to intensify health and nutrition education efforts, but also to establish, through the mothers' clubs, a system of distribution of foods at lower prices than those in the market. This would allow the gradual phasing out of free-of-charge food supplies and ensure the continuation of the programme at the end of external assistance. Furthermore, the Government intends to stimulate the mothers' clubs to undertake cooperative productive activities and thus contribute to the integration of women in their own community and therefore in the overall development process of the country.

11. CONCLUSION

This paper has tried to spell out a particular problem area for maternal and child health, and to suggest some solutions. There remains, however, several missing ingredients. Perhaps we have overemphasized the negative aspects of particular cases to make our point. Certainly, not enough is known about how the different kinds of institutional arrangements work out in practice. And not enough is known about the specific, and most appropriate support measures which these institutions need. There is a need then for action research in this area which will prepare the way for more effective strategies. Finally, there is the need to communicate this information more widely so that many countries can draw on the experience of others, whether this is positive or negative. It is in this process of communication that the international agencies can play a vital role in pointing the way to more rationally integrated food distribution and the improvement of maternal and child health.

APPENDIX I

NUTRITION SUPPLEMENTARY PROGRAMME IN INDIA*
A REASSESSMENT

Malnutrition never occurs in isolation. It is a result of adverse socio-economic and poor educational status, deep rooted cultural beliefs, poor environmental sanitation and unsatisfactory water supply with its resultant high prevalence of infections, particularly diarrhoeal disorders. Malnutrition is a major contributory cause of death between the age of 1 month and 2 years in all developing countries and unless these children can be benefited from a nutrition programme and the morbidity can be reduced, the usefulness of the programme could be questioned. The nutrition supplement programmes have been in operation for the past many years, with an outlay of 3000-4000 million rupees in the Vth plan period. The Poshak Project of CARE while establishing the feasibility of such a programme, failed to produce any significant nutritional benefits. Milk given out in urban MCH centres has damaged an excellent tradition of breast-feeding resulting in infections and malnutrition. Reckless distribution of skimmed milk in the past actually increased the incidence of keratomalacia and blindness in some regions. The time of the health workers was spent in distributing powdered milk to mothers, with no time to observe, diagnose, treat or advise. Often the milk was used for the family tea with no benefit to the child. The beneficiary at best looked upon it as a little saving of money rather than a nutrition supplement. When the milk supply stopped, the mothers stopped coming.

*Shanti Ghosh

Even where it is a part of a more comprehensive programme such as the ICDS* Programme, almost half of the time of the workers is spent in cooking, distributing the food and cleaning up afterwards, rather than spending the time in health and nutrition education, non-formal education health care etc. The attention of the Anganwadi workers, the supervisors, and the administrators is focussed on the nutrition supplement part of the programme and everything else tends to get neglected, and so there can be no returns in the form of better health, lower morbidity and lower mortality. The nutrition supplement thus remains the most expensive part of this programme and the problem in sheer logistics is staggering.

Institutional feeding programme as looked upon in its proper perspective has its uses. In schools, the children are away from their homes for 5-6 hours and so a mid-day meal programme would be sensible and useful provided it supplied better quality food than the child would have normally brought from home. It should be palatable, have some variety and should be nutritious. It also should have an element of nutrition education which the child can carry home, such as the importance of green vegetables, better methods of cooking advantages of sprouted vegetables etc. It has to be accepted that the meal is a substitute for the home food rather than a "do good" programme for better nutrition. It is invariably a substitution and not an addition to the child's food. The same would apply to a preschool programme. Some children have no appetite for the kind of food offered. As one child said, "The gutters were running white with lumps of it". The death rate in this group is high and malnutrition is an important underlying cause. These children are never seen at any food supplement centre. The reason

* Infant and Child Development Services

for their malnutrition is not so much the lack of food but the child's dependence on his mother who has no knowledge of his nutritional needs and so does not feed him. This can only be solved by nutrition education and demonstration at an individual level and not by food supplement.

What is needed therefore is emphasis on health and nutrition education through properly trained local workers who are in turn supervised by better trained health workers. For it to have any impact, the vehicle of nutrition education should be the locally produced food preferably contributed by villagers themselves. No outside food can achieve that. This has to be integrated with the total health care programme where the prevention and treatment of morbidity (which is the most important felt need) has to be taken care of. The worker population ratio also would have to be more realistic if any results have to be achieved.

Food supplements are justified in certain situations such as emergencies like floods, droughts etc. which naturally will be time bound and target oriented, as a temporary measure in a scarcity area, again time bound and target oriented, institutionalised feeding as described earlier and at an individual level where the breastmilk has failed or where there is a temporary family deprivation due to unemployment, death etc.

The causes of undernutrition are mainly economical, social and cultural. A solution therefore cannot be expected from health measures, leave alone a nutrition supplement. They are at the most palliative and have a limited effect. Full integration of nutrition activities with other health activities, is necessary. Nutrition supplement should be looked at as a hard cost benefit accounting exercise. Investments in better water supply and sewage disposal, better facility for primary health care within 1-2 km radius, training local workers in primary health care, improving the worker population ratio and use of indigenous medical facilities wherever feasible is likely to produce much better dividends than food distribution. Time has therefore come to have a second look at the nutrition supplement programmes and do some serious thinking as to whether these resources both in money and manpower cannot be better utilised in the main job of reducing deaths to malnutrition and infections.

APPENDIX II

COMMENTS ON THE PAPER*

Evidence shows that food distribution programs have had considerable benefits, although in many cases it may have been below the expected level.Our review of the Indian experience(2) confirmed program benefits at varying levels. However, the sum total of the Indian experience seems to be better than pictured in this paper.

In a good number of cases food collection seems to be the primary purpose of referring to the MCH centers. If so, then that is a positive indication of a strong-felt need for more food in the household. This is quite contrary to the statement made in the paper that the reason for malnutrition is not so much lack of food but the child's dependence on an illiterate mother.

It would be extemely useful if the MCH centers actively screen the needy child for food assistance. Such careful targeting would allow for more efficient use of food for the real needy. Unfortunately screening is given very little attention at these centers at present. Once screening is made, then food collection needs to be made within a conveniently accessible point. If possible to arrange for food collection outside the center it would be quite satisfactory. However, there is strong reason for concern in the areas where the outreach and institutional arrangements are extremely limited. Traditionally health infrastructure has better

*H. Ghassemi - 26.3.81.

outreach in many places. It is well understood that food distribution should not be entirely the responsibility of the professional staff. Wherever it happens it is due to poor management and inadequate division of responsibilities rather than the value of food for vulnerable individuals.

There is increasing interest and emphasis on integration of community services. There is substantial evidence that food and health care together will do better than each provided separately. If so, then taking food distribution out of the health system seems to be getting away from the integration concept.

As stated in Appendix I on Indian experiences, undernutrition can often be due to economical problems, e.g. family is extremely poor, there is not enough food in the house, and the young child is very likely to receive less than his fair share of the food available. Under the conditions of severe poverty and tight food situation, one effective way to narrow the food gap would be to provide food for the poor household. It is agreed that food distribution is a palliative measure. However, if the child is hungry because of lack of enough food then it will be hard to argue that immunization and sanitation can effectively serve as a substitute. Under such circumstances food distribution may be looked at as one way to close the food gap.

However, it is true that in many occasions food may not reach the needy; as a matter of fact, it may be given to the least needy. Identification of the hungry as against the adequately fed or marginally underfed is necessary.

Dissatisfaction with feeding may be for one or more of the following reasons:

a) food is not adequate in quantity and/or quality (inadequate programming);

b) food does not reach the needy (inadequate implementation);

c) benefits may not be adequately measured, e.g. did not look at the increased physical activity (inadequate evaluation).

FOOTNOTES

(1) For a balanced review see Jonathan Fryer - 1981 - Food for Thought - The Use and Abuse of Food Aid in the Fight Against World Hunger - WCC-Geneva See also Singir H.W. - 1980 - Food Aid Policies & Programmes - Food & Nutrition Bulletin, V.2,No.3.

(2) For a basically positive view see Beaton E.H. & Ghasseni H. - 1979 - Supplementary Feeding Programmes for Young Children in Developing Countries - UNICEF. This has also some notes on improving programme effectiveness.

CHAPTER FIVE

SELF RELIANCE IN AN URBAN SQUATTER SETTLEMENTS-
SANG KANCIL: KUALA LUMPUR, MALAYSIA

This paper describes the situation of communities in squatter settlements in Kuala Lumpur, and how they managed through self reliance to improve their own health and cooperated with the agencies. The project was named Sang Kancil, after the tiny mouse deer in the Malaysian jungle. This tiny creature relies on clever ideas to survive as people in urban slums must also do.

Statistics on squatter settlements are sensitive issues. Data on distribution, age-specific population groups and dimensions of squatter areas and ethnic composition are not readily obtainable, until very recently. Squatter settlements by its very nature are unlawful settlements. The high concentration of the urban poor group; in an underdeveloped small land mass creates a political and social dilemma for the authorities.

The affluent Kuala Lumpurians who daily commute to work in air-conditioned cars, to make life more bearable in the traffic jam, do not realise that hidden behind high rise buildings, banks, government offices, lies the largest squatter population in the country.

Squatter settlements usually arise spontaneously, almost overnight, and proliferate quickly by the further addition of squatter houses usually within a period of months. The total households in each squatter settlement varies between 300 - 1,500. Many of the settlements have a population between 1,000 - 8,000 people. The rapidity with which a squatter community develops is vital to the survival of the community itself because with increase in numbers, leadership structures can be formed, which will then try to strengthen the fledgling settlement and prevent it from being dismantled by City Hall. With the recent formation of an enforcement unit, City Hall is able to contain the proliferation of squatter settlements in Kuala Lumpur. For those settlements which survive it is vital that some kind of outside assistance be mobilised to protect its communities. One of the very important functions of its leaders is to seek assistance from strong personages, prominent individuals, political organisations and ultimately to establish loyalty and allegiance to specific organisations.

The association of squatter communities with political groups has given the squatter communities much needed help and impetus to obtain the basic necessities for survival, such as water stand pipes, sanitation, garbage clearance, drainage, and to a limited extent access roads. As the settlements gain in strength and self assurance, demands for basic amenities become more vociferous and insistent;

which all too frequently cause conflicts between those who oversee long term planning in sanitation, licensing and highways. A compromise is therefore necessary between squatters and City Hall, the latter deprived of specific socio-political guidelines will provide just sufficient basic amenities for garbage disposal, sanitation and water stand pipes, without committing itself to heavy infrastructure development such as buildings, electricity, telephone lines and individual water supply. How much is enough is a source of conflict between City Hall and squatters, who are only too well aware that they are occupying unlawfully a piece of expensive real estate. The source of conflict will remain unless a firm socio-political decision is made not only on squatting but on ethnic composition of urban cities, entrepreneurship, distribution of business opportunities among ethnic groups and policy on population distribution.

The solution to squatter problems in Malaysia has to be taken in the context of the socio-political climate of the country. Currently City Hall is trying to solve some of the more acute squatter problems by:

a) the restriction of further expansion of illegal dwellings

b) the provision of "longhouses" as a transit camps for those who have to be moved to high rise flats

c) upgrading of selected settlements into a permanent urban development centre by providing legal title and deeds for each dwelling

There was an uneasiness at such an approach where recommendations were directed from the "top" by groups of planners some of whom may not even have seen a squatter settlement. Assumptions by those who have had wide experience of delivering health services to the rural areas, erroneously concluded that the requirements are probably the same as in a rural community. However, it was decided that these assumptions should be tested.

The methods used to test assumptions of needs were by:

(i) A Base Line Study

(ii) Dialogue with communities

(iii) "Berbual" informal unstructured interaction with mothers and husbands at various time and places convenient to the interviewee

(iv) Interview of communities leaders

(i) <u>Base Line Study</u>

Information on basic needs were extracted from census data made available by City Hall on the three pilot study areas, namely Kampong Abdullah Hukom, Kampong Malaysia Tambahan and Kampong Pandan.

The three communities felt their most important basic needs were water and electricity. An important health factor such as garbage disposal was not even a major issue. A clinic health centre was not as important as recreational halls and telephones. The importance of health facilities did not clearly manifest itself and the strategy of delivering health care as a major intervention programme clearly needed to be reassessed.

Based on the concept of communities need, it seemed clear that the emphasis on health should now be redirected to the provision of water supply, electricity, telephone and recreation halls. But it was also realised that such an intervention programme will be difficult to get off the ground since these issues are long standing and not easily resolved because of political overtones and the difficulties of intersectoral co-ordination. The apparent basic needs of the squatters themselves have to be re-examined and a compromise will have to be reached. The following describes how compromise was reached.

(ii) Dialogue with Communities

Meetings with squatters who reside on the three pilot areas were held several times to establish the "true need" of the communities, to explain the objectives of Sang Kancil and to assess reaction of the communities towards the proposed programme.

The general feelings of the squatter communities during such dialogue was one of polite acceptance. It seemed that many such meetings have been held before by other project implementers.

The hidden consensus was that Sang Kancil will probably not proceed beyond the "talking stage". But initial reservation was slowly overcome as the project takes shape. With subsequent dialogue and consultations mutual trust and respect were established, and the planners reaffirmed that the Sang Kancil Programme would not be forced upon them if there were wide feelings of dissatisfactions. The community was reassured also that the project will be established quickly.

During the early learning process of communication with the squatters it was noted that the discussions were ususally dominated by individuals with strong personalities, who may or may not reflect the needs of the majority, who because of shyness, ignorance and illiteracy, choose to remain silent. But successful programmes will depend on the support of this silent majority. Psychological barriers to free communication with the silent majority, may arise as a result of improper technique such as in the choice of words, ability to accept the squatters on equal terms and most importantly the ability to project an image of sincerity and the avoidance of a condescending attitude on part of the planners. However, not all planners have these skills.

A better method of communication has to be found.

(iii) <u>"Berbual"</u>

Of the many methods used, "berbual" is the most sensitive technique of establishing needs even if it suffers somewhat from scientific objectivity and general acceptibility of expression of the community.

"Berbual" is a Bahasa Malaysia term which describes a set pattern of behaviour by which groups or individuals talk to each other. It has an implied sense of democracy where both parties are treated as equal. Ranks are usually forgotten. Informality is the order of the day. Both parties are relaxed. Serious business are preceded usually by inconsequential subject matter.

This technique was used effectively to reinforce understanding on the needs of the squatters. The time for "berbual" takes account of the subjects availabilitiy. For mothers in the morning while they are washing clothes, at the stand pipes or at home preparing the day's work. Beside the demand for basic amenities there is a consistent request for pre-school education. Both parents believe that education is the key issue for their children to break the cycle of poverty.

Others were even of the opinion that the centres may not be such a good idea as it will take away the only free play ground available for their children.

Some squatters suggested that the space occupied by the houses rented by squatters were owned by "affluent people who live outside" the kampong. They felt the space could be used for the centre.

General consensus by the squatters were that many promised projects take too long to be implemented, so that after a while it lowered the credibility of the implementers.

(iv) Interview with Squatter Leaders

The leadership structures of the squatter settlements are complex. Generally they consist of:

1. Leaders who are members of political organisations
2. Leaders who are selected because of strong personality
3. Religious Leaders
4. The elders
5. Penghulus (appointed by government)
6. Old midwives

It was important to establish communication with the "real" leaders. Some leaders motivated by personal advancement will support programmes which may be in conflict with the real needs of the communities. The desire to please authorities in order to strengthen their individual power will not achieve long term support by the majority of the community.

An interesting phenomenon in leadership structure is the selection of leaders who do not live in the squatter settlements themselves. Conflicts and disenchantment usually occurs under such a situation. Generally, such persons may not be recognised as the true leader of the community.

Leaders from political organisations also play important roles. Political organisations usually arise spontaneously in squatter communities. The leadership position usually enables direct access to Members of Parliament and Ministers. The leader is able to bring problems to higher authorities who in turn will exert pressure on the implementing agency. However, sometimes such ad hoc measures are not always conducive for long term planning for programme implementers. For instance, a squatter may demand to have extra stand pipes brought to his kampong and the proper agency will be directed to fulfil this request. But because of lack of coordination and understanding on the role of the agency concerned, and through no fault of its own, the water stand pipe will be built but no water will be channelled because of lack of water pressure in the area.

The dialogue with leaders of the three pilot areas was to ensure full participation and co-operation from the community. The project will not gain ground if the leaders are hostile.

But generally the leader themselves have been sympathetic and have given their utmost support and co-operation for the project - although this may not initially be shared by the rest of the squatters. Experience has shown that initial enthusiasm alone does not last unless the project is quickly put on the ground.

Administrative Organisation

After these discussions a unit was established within the framework of the City Hall administrative structure to implement the Sang Kancil Programme. It is assisted by a small technical group of members with specific skills. From past experience it was realised that large committees do not necessarily contribute to the efficiency, quality and speed of implementation of the project. The members were:

1. Director-General of City Hall (Chairman)
2. Director of Development and Co-ordination (Project Manager)
3. Medical Officer of City Hall (Overall supervision of MCH clinic)
4. Matron of Nursing Service of City Hall (Supervisor of MCH clinics)
5. Assistant Director of MCH from Ministry of Health
6. Supervisor of Pre-school Education from KEMAS (Government Agency on Community Development
7. Executive Officer of National Unity Board
8. Honorary Consultant of Sang Kancil (Professor of Social Obstetric and Gynaecology, University of Malaya

Aims of Sang Kancil

Based on information of preliminary study and as a result of interaction with the community, it was decided that pre-school education had much higher priorities than a maternal and child health clinic and that it should be established first.

Accordingly the Sang Kancil Programme established a specified series of aims in which maternal and child health was incorporated as part of human development, recognising that it is secondary to other important perceptions of needs, which are pre-school education and income generating activities. From the planner's point of view it was realised that community participation should also be incorporated as an important component of Sang Kancil (Chart.1).

1. To develop a centre within each squatter community to enable planners, institutional resources and medical personnel to be easily accessible to the beneficiaries. To identify and solve problems and needs of the community in an environment which is conducive and non-threatening to the beneficiaries.

2. to provide health services for mother and child based on clinic settings.

3. To develop pre-school activities as a means of community participation and to establish contact with central childcare giver, so that appropriate interaction can be established between planners and the family on problems of the growing child.

4. To identify and strengthen community participation by incorporating community leaders in the decision making process and to plan activities which necessitate assistance from the beneficiaries; for example in pre-school education mothers have to assist pre-school teachers on their environmental trips as field assistants; participation of community leaders in planning and selection of pre-school community teachers and the training of women for income generating activities.

Chart 1

SANG KANCIL PRIMARY HEALTH CARE SYSTEM FOR URBAN SQUATTERS

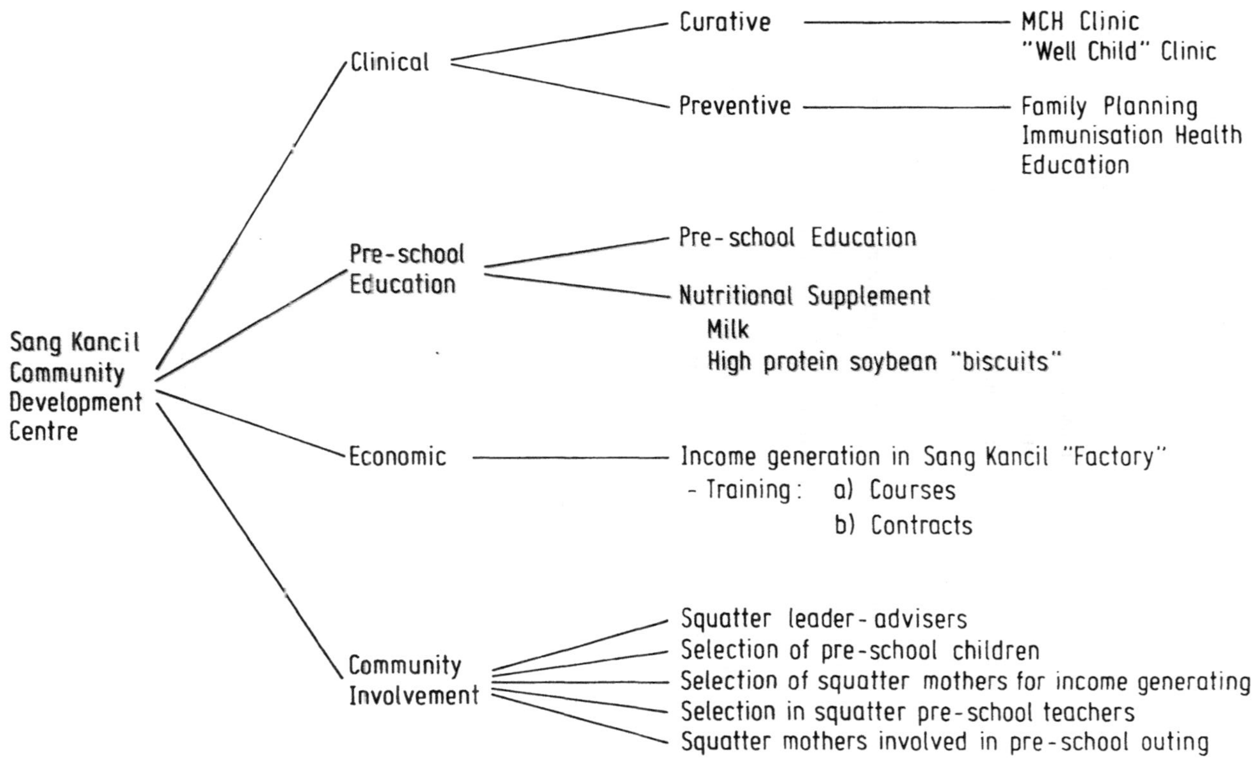

5. To develop a system for income generating activities in order to fulfill the perceived and apparent needs of the community.

6. To develop and train specific manpower needs of the Sang Kancil Programme based on existing resources such as the community pre-school teachers from squatter women, and Nurse-Practitioners for Mother and Child from City Hall nurses.

7. To use the Sang Kancil Programme for the training of:
   a) Medical students at University Hospital, in Social Obstetrics and Gynaecology.

   (b) Government servants in communication, to heighten sensitivity and awareness on the need of the urban poor.

8. To generate multidisciplinary social research activities on urban squatters and to monitor the social and economic changes in the settlements.

Physical Facilities of Sang Kancil

Critical to the Sang Kancil concept was the construction of a building centrally located in the squatter settlements itself. This is intended to provide easy accessibility for the community and hence greater incentive to participate in income generating activities, pre-school education and the utilisation of the MCH clinic services. (See Fig. 2)

Fig. 2
PHYSICAL STRUCTURE OF SANG KANCIL
(Kampong Malaysia Tambahan)

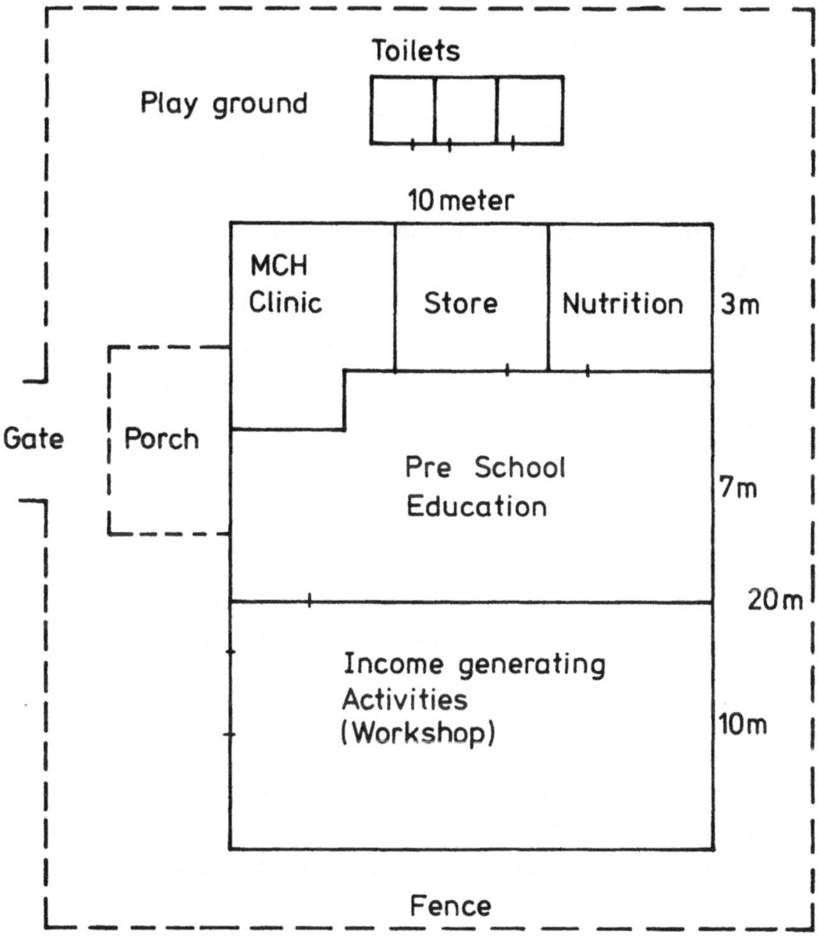

It is also hoped that the obvious physical visibility of the centre within the community will in time give a sense of proprietorship to the community and hence to inspire community sense of commitment and participation. It has not been easy to implement this concept since squatter houses by tradition are built closely grouped together.

The City Hall (Development and Co-ordinating Unit) has been the prime force in establishing the buildings of these two pilot project areas. Funds and materials were quickly made available and with the staff knowledge of existing land space, the buildings were erected within 10-14 months respectively, a remarkable achievement considering the long drawn out process which is required normally to set up a building by a government agency. In the case of Sang Kancil the cost of the building is comparatively small, much of the bureaucratic machinery has been bypassed.

Manpower Requirements for Sang Kancil

It was recognised early on during the preparatory stage of Sang Kancil that there was a need to develop an internal manpower resource, in the area of health and pre-school education. It will not be possible for City Hall to recruit doctors to manage the various Sang Kancil Clinics in the squatter areas which will be expanded to a total of 20 centres by 1985. One of the main reasons is due to the movement of doctors to the more lucrative private sectors. But the drift of doctors from public to private sectors does not imply that the urban poor will benefit. Firstly, most of the urban poor cannot afford private medical service. Secondly, many of the clinics are located in the more prosperous areas where they are accessible to middle class clienteles.

The concept of nurse-practitioner (mother and child) as key personnel for delivery of primary health care was developed to overcome the medical manpower shortage for the programme. The MCH clinics will cater only for mother and child in an attempt to deliver health services to the most vulnerable numbers of the family. The narrowing of health care will enable limited manpower and financial resources to be more efficiently utilised.

Income Generating Activities

The concept of income generating activities was developed under the same roof with pre-school education and MCH clinics. It is perhaps the most difficult part of the programme to implement. The idea of training squatter housewives in specific skills to supplement their income is not new, especially among women. But in Malaysia there has been no attempt to apply this concept among squatter women. But after courses a succesful tailoring enterprise was established. The increase in monthly cash income combined with proper consumer education will have a far reaching effect on the general health of the family. Health education on nutrition for instance will only have limited value to the poor families who cannot even afford the basic necessities of life. Unlike their rural counterparts land is unavailable to the urban poor for home grown vegetable gardens, and for the raising of domestic animals. The usual response to health education on nutrition is the inability to buy necessary food for the family due to rising cost of basic staple diet such as vegetables and fish. The income generating activity shows promise in that it will assist the squatter mothers to overcome some of these problems.

Income generating activities also acknowledge the express priority of the beneficiary. The overall impetus of development of the programme may in the long run be restricted unless the basic need of the community is recognised. By establishing a Sang Kancil "factory" along side pre-school and health clinics, the programme implementers accept and recognise the fact that the main problems of the squatters are not entirely due to health and pre-school education.

Sang Kancil and Intersectoral Co-ordination

One of the tenets of primary health care is to seek improvement of those factors which have direct association to health, such as nutrition, education, sanitation, water supply, personal health care, control of diseases vectors and mass immunisation. The use of simultaneous multipronged approach has never been tested among squatter communities of Malaysia. It is unlikely to achieve similar success as in rural areas, because squatter communities are in fact illegal settlements. Unless basic political decisions are made to change the unlawful status, as is being done in a few squatter settlements of Kuala Lumpur i.e. Kampong Malaysia Tambahan, and Kampong Kongo, basic health saving measures such as water supply, proper sanitation, electricity and refuse disposal cannot be provided except in a retroactive manner.

Sang Kancil and Community Participation

Community participation is well defined and explicit in the Sang Kancil Programme. These are the involvement of mothers in pre-school activities, decision making and assistance in selection of community pre-school teachers, assistance in planning and participation in income generating activities. Squatter settlements have tightly knit, intimate social and hierachial leadership structures. The existence of Sang Kancil within the midst of small catchment areas has in a psychological sense created an atmosphere for easier community involvement which can be measured and observed from the planner's and community's point of view. For instance individuals and committees who have been delegated certain jobs are strongly motivated to carry it out with credit because they will be closely judged by their peer groups and neighbours.

The loss of face is a strong incentive. This cultural idiosyncracy can be used effectively to improve community participation. Similarly as beneficiary the squatter themselves can also judge the ability of the planners to deliver the goods and promises.

CONCLUSION

The Sang Kancil Programme has been in operation for three years. On-going evaluation based on interviews of squatter women and based on perceptions by planners and international visitors, seems to indicate that the programme is developing in a way which is most encouraging. Evaluation of the preschool education has supported this and the health activitites which have been implemented by nurse-practitioners have shown the benefits of having a clinic almost at the door-steps of the beneficiaries. The narrowing of health care to children and to the health of the mother has kept the programme manageable. However, the learning process for both planners and beneficiaries does not seem to stop even at this late stage because problems do appear in different forms, guises and from different directions. There is a never ending interaction, understanding and learning by both parties. Lessons learnt from Sang Kancil are that human problems and conflicts do not come in neat packages to be solved one at a time.

With the successful implementation of the pilot projects, the Sang Kancil Programme has been accepted by the Malaysian Government as one of the means to help the urban poor through a holistic system of health care deliveries. A total of 20 centres are planned and have been accepted in the 4th Malaysia Plan. Five more centres will have been added in 1981 and the rest will be implemented within the next three years.

It is relevant perhaps to emphasise that when the Sang Kancil Programme expands to 20 centres covering a population of 100,000 squatters the capabilities of the planners will be tested. Motivation, enthusiasm and administrative infrastructure will be stretched to the utmost and the problems encountered will be far greater than those which the planners had faced during the period of testing.

CHAPTER SIX

MATERNAL AND CHILD HEALTH IN WESTERN SAMOA

AN INTERSECTORAL VIEW*

1. INTRODUCTION

Demographers, geographers, planners in health and development - all varieties of "experts" visit Western Samoa and invariably ask the same question. "How do you account for the relatively low infant mortality rate (IMR), when you apparently have a low gross national product (GNP) per capita?"

It is believed that Western Samoa's national income per capita is around US$ 350, a large proportion being from subsistence production which is consumed directly by households. Despite the low GNP, Samoa's designation as one of the world's "least developed nations" and despite complaints of the declining standard of living, one is still impressed by the relative abundance of food, the absence of visible suffering from disease, widespread distribution of consumer goods and improved housing and village schools.

* Paper prepared by Viopapa Annandale, Rula Levi and Iuni Sapolu

To what extent if at all, do these favourable attributes affect the status of health of women and children in Samoa and how have these levels of development been reached? This paper is an attempt to present a realistic and critical look at the situation of maternal and child health (MCH) and will discuss the dynamics of this situation.

2. BACKGROUND INFORMATION

2.1 Geographic and ethnic characteristics:

Western Samoa is a small independent island nation, situated in the South Pacific. The population estimated at 160,000 in mid-year 1979, live on four of the islands, mainly in villages scattered along coastal areas. About 60% reside on the island of Upolu, where the capital city of Apia is situated. Around 25% of the total population live in Apia, and not surprisingly this ratio is increasing each year. The construction of many access roads have made it possible for many families to settle and to develop lands inland from the coast.

The population is ethnically homogeneous, the majority being full or part Polynesian. The few other ethnic groups are well assimilated. Christianity is almost universally practised in Samoa.

There are few natural resources and the export earnings do not meet the escalating costs of increasing dependency on imported consumer goods. The shifting dependency on a cash economy has had expected effects on family health and Samoan family life.

2.2 The Political System

The country is governed by a Cabinet of Ministers, chosen and headed by a Prime Minister, who is elected by the Members of Parliament. Samoa is divided into forty-three (43) political constituencies, each of which are represented in Parliament by one member. Only chiefs or title holders (matais) are eligible to stand for election and to vote for their representative. Thus the people do not enjoy universal suffrage, except for a small minority of the population of mixed ethnic descent who are not under the matai system. This group is represented by two members who are elected by universal suffrage.

2.3. Health Services

Health services are provided through a three-tiered system. At the grass-roots or community level the District Nurses serving an average of 3,000 people provide mainly preventive and follow-up care. There are 14 health districts, each with a small District Hospital, to which the people attend for secondary level of health care. These hospitals are staffed by a District Medical Officer (DMO), Staff Nurses and a number of ancillary staff depending on their availability. Due to the chronic shortage of medical manpower not all districts have a DMO. Complicated or serious cases are referred to the National Hospital in Apia, which has about 311 beds. The National Hospital is currently being rebuilt and modernised and provides reasonably modern medical investigative and specialist curative services. It also serves the population of Apia for primary health care. As in most developing countries, there is some inequity with the distribution of health manpower but the present Government is committed to the Primary Health Care concept and high priority is given to meeting the health needs of the rural population.

In-patients and Out-patients pay a very minimal fee for services. During the last 4 years, a few doctors have started private practice, but they are almost exclusively concentrated in the Apia urban area.

The skills and influence of traditional healers is not clearly defined, but it is believed that traditional healers play an important role in the health of Samoan families, especially the Traditional Birth Attendants (TBA) who attend about 40-50% of all deliveries. A short course for around 400 TBA's was conducted during 1976 and 1977.

3. SELECTED INDICATORS OF MATERNAL AND CHILD HEALTH

The usual accepted indicators of maternal and child health (MCH) are not easy to analyse as existing information collection and reporting systems are inadequate. Report forms currently being used by the Department of Health are complicated. What information that are reported are often incomplete and unreliable, and oriented more towards indices of performance rather than towards outcome or impact of the services. Furthermore, accurate baseline population data at the district level are not complete.

The difficulty is compounded even further by the fact that different government departments publish different sets of statistics, and we are often surprised to find a separate set again, being published by international agencies such as the World Bank and the U.N. The picture is therefore confused. For consistency we have decided to refer mainly to the Health Statistics for Western Samoa - 1979, published by the Department of Health, and where necessary will compare this source with other sources.

3.1 Crude Birth Rate and Total Fertility Rate

Th registered number of births in 1979 was 2,889 i.e. a crude birth rate (CBR) of 18.3/1000 population. The Department of Statistics in the Annual Statistical Abstract for 1979 published an estimated CBR in 1979 of 33.5/1000 population. The Fourth Five Year Development Plan, for Western Samoa, 1980-1984, Vol.1 gives a CBR for 1979 (page 13) of 37.4/1000. From the general population census (1971-1976) it was found that the CBR was between 37-38/1000.

We are of the opinion that the CBR is now somewhere in the region of 35/1000 and base our calculations on this variable.

In 1969 the registered number of births was 4330, a drop of registered births by 33% in 10 years. Was the decline really to this extent? We think not, and suggest that the system for reporting births needs great improvement. It was estimated by the Family Welfare Section, after the last Family Planning Current User Survey conducted in September 1980, that approximately 15% of the eligible female population (15-49 years) were using a family planning method. The apparently rapid decline in registered births during the last 10 years cannot be accounted for by high use of birth control methods.

It is an interesting finding that since 1956, census reports have consistently shown that more boys are born than girls. The sex ratio is 110 males to 100 females, a ratio believed to be the highest in the world!

The total Fertility Rate calculated from census of population for the period 1966-1971 was estimated at 7.4. During the subsequent period of 1971-1976 it declined to 6.7.

As might be expected the CBR and TFR for the Apia Urban Area is lower than those for other areas. (See table 1 below)

Table 1: Total Fertility Rates and Crude Birth Rates
Four Regions - Samoa
1971 - 1976

Region	Total Fertility Rate	Crude Birth Rate
Apia Urban Area	5.5	33.7
North West Upolu	6.9	37.3
Rest of Upolu	7.4	18.0
Savaii	6.9	37.5

Source: Census of population and housing, 1976, Analytical Report, p.76 Vol. 2

3.2 Infant Mortality Rate (IMR)

Once again we find a confusing picture. In 1979 there were only 51 reported infant deaths i.e an IMR of 17.6/1000 live births - comparable to a developed country: In 1969 there were 120 reported infant deaths. It is clear that reliable rates cannot be calculated from the civil registration system or from the reporting system of the Health Department.

According to the Analytical Report Vol. 2, of the Census of Population and Housing 1976, Western Samoa has a surprisingly low infant mortality. The infant mortality rate is about 36/1000 live births, which is considered to be much less than the demographers expect on the basis of current life expectancies. The Western Samoa life table for 1971-1976 shows that the life expectancy were for males 60 years and for females 63 years. There has been a slight increase for the two sexes over the previous 5-10 years. If we were to compare the life expectancies of Samoa with those appearing in the model life tables, the IMR would be close to 50/1000 life births! This apparently means that the infant mortality to Western Samoa is lower than indicated by mortality experience from a broad number of countries used for deriving the model life tables (Analytical Report Vol. 2).

Of the reported 51 infant deaths in 1979, 39.2% died within the first week of life, and 47.1% by the first month. No causes of death are published nor are there figures to indicate foetal wastage. This high proportion of neonatal deaths indicate the need for better antenatal, natal and immediate post-natal care. The most likely cause of death of 1-11 month old (again unpublished) are respiratory diseases, diarrhoel diseases and possibly from complications from measles and in association with malnutrition.

3.3 Infant and Child Morbidity

There are no published data available on infant and child morbidity other than for infantile diarrhoea. The incidence of reported cases in 1970 was 1736.5/100.000 population, and in 1979 had dropped to 542.3/100.000. It is likely that with improved supply of potable water and excreta disposal, the actual number has really declined. (80% of the population have easy access to clean water and 71% use recommended excreta disposal units, mainly in the form of water seal latrines.)

Other statistics on morbidity are not age specific. Respiratory tract infections, middle ear infections, malnutrition, diarrhoel diseases, and communicable diseases such as measles, chicken-pox and occasionally whooping cough are considered to be the most common causes of infant and child morbidity. Parasitic infestation and skin infections are widespread and bothersome.

Early childhood malnutrition is increasing. A WHO study conducted by Dr. A.A. Janssen in 1969 showed that 4.6% of a sample size of 2,261 infants had mild to moderate signs of malnutrition. Of the 2 year olds, 11.7% were malnourished, and of the 3 year olds, 10.9%. The overall rate for children aged 0-5 years (sample size 3,933) was 6.9%.

An interesting shift was demonstrated in another study conducted in 1979 by an Australian Volunteer Social Worker, Helen Brazill. Ms. Brazill found that 33% of her sample of infants (253) were malnourished. The shift may have been due to some bias in her sampling methods. The overall malnutrition rate of a total of 972 children aged 0-3 years was 19.5%.

The problem of early childhood protein-energy malnutrition (PEM) today is essentially a problem associated with a transitional social and economic phase of development. Children living on the island of Savaii are apparently least affected.

In 1980 a second WHO study confirmed that PEM among preschool children has increased considerably during the decade 1969-1979. The childhood mortality rate from PEM is not known since infants who die are usually reported as having died from complications or associated secondary conditions arising from malnutrition.

The main causes of early childhood malnutrition stems from the increasing incidence of artificial feeding and early weaning, either as a result of frequent childbearing, adoption (a fairly widespread practice in Samoa), early return to paid employment or poor knowledge or understanding or proper infant feeding practices. Samoan culture places children low in the pecking order but this is not considered to be a major contributing factor of PEM. There is no shortage of food in Samoa, but poor distribution of what is available particularly to low-income families can be another important contributing factor.

3.4 Coverage of Child Health/Services

An evaluative study of the MCH project carried out by the Family Welfare Section (responsible for MCH & FP) of the Health Department in September 1980 showed a very encouraging improvement in the overall coverage of child health care. In 1976 it was found that an average of 55% of infants (0-11 months) and 66% of pre-schoolers (1-4 years) had a current Child Health Record. The results in 1980 was 81.4% and 72.6% respectively. A good proportion of those children had received regular assessments of weight and of growth and development.

It is surprising therefore to find that the percentage of children with completed immunisations (DPTTY, Polio and BCG) was a low 27% in 1976 and 43.8% in 1980. An EPI project has just began in Western Samoa and it is expected that coverage for immunisation will improve greatly. Measles vaccine is now added to the vaccines given, and the typhoid component has been dropped.

3.5 Maternal morbidity and mortality

One maternal death was reported in 1979 i.e. a maternal death rate of 0.3/1000 live births: The reported rates have been consistently low during the last few years which suggests persistent under-reporting. The crude death rate (from all causes) based on reported events has remained around 3.5/1000 population during recent years. The estimated CDR, however is in the region of 7.5/1000 population annually.

Causes of maternal death are not reported and it is not possible to find published reports of causes of maternal morbidity. The Head of the Obstetrics and Gynaecology Unit of the National Hospital however is of the opinion that hypertensive diseases of pregnancy, urinary tract infections and antepartum or postpartum haemorrhage are the main causes of maternal morbidity in patients seen in Apia.

3.6 Other indicators of maternal health

One of the indicators studies, during the evaluative study of the MCH project mentioned earlier, was the percentage of pregnant women attending ante-natal clinic at least once. It was found that by far the majority of pregnant women attended twice or more, and that over 100% of pregnant women in Apia received antenatal care and around 80% of rural women. Unfortunately, however, the average gestational age of the foetus at first visit was 25 weeks.

There hase been attempts to investigate average blood haemoglobin levels of pregnant women who attend antenatal clinic. From two small studies recently conducted, the haemoglobin level was found to lie between 108 and 11.4mgs/100 mls. WHO has suggested that the haemoglobin concentration below which anaemia is likely to be present at sea-level for pregnant women is 11 mgs/100 mls.

Recorded birth weights of infants born in the National Hospital in 1979 show that 37.2% had birth weigths between 3180-3600 grams (a somewhat odd grouping!) and 25.6% had weights below 3180 grams. It should be noted that the National Hospital serves as a referral centre for the whole country and therefore it is not surprising that the average birth weight would tend to be on the low side. It is our impression from examining a large number of child health records both in Apia and in rural areas of Upolu and Savaii, that at least 50% of newborns weigh 3500 grams or more at birth.

Because of gross under-reporting of births it is again uncertain what proportion of infants are delivered by trained personnel. The Health Department published statistics for 1979 stating that 81% of births are delivered in a hospital, but from examining child health records, we found that 41.4% of infants with records in Rural Upolu and 66% in Savaii were delivered by TBA's. It is because of this high proportion that the Department of Health plans to examine more closely the possibility to retrain TBA's not only to improve their midwifery practice, but to provide a broader scope of mother and child care.

4. THE DYNAMICS: CAUSAL AND CONTRIBUTING FACTORS

4.1 Cultural Factors

The culture of Samoa is noted for its relative resistance to foreign influence. What has changed, resulted from a gradual blending and molding of palagi (foreign) ways and thinking into the Samoan. Overall, we believe that the cultural and traditional attitudes and practices of Samoa have a net positive effect on health. Problems, however, have arisen from conflicts created by some aspects of development, which is necessarily associated with foreign influence.

These conflicts are best described to the words of an elderly village woman.
"The health of women and children in Samoa does not depend on money. Money has made people selfish and driven the most able people of my village to poorly paid jobs in town leaving children in the care of old people like myself. I cannot look after four youngsters, two of whom are toddlers. I cannot make a saka (boiled food). Someone else has to look after the children."

Another middle-aged nurse believes that "sophisticated health programs are impossible without observing cultural rules and practices that thave existed and are still existing in the community". This illustrates the need to consider new health ideas in the context of existing cultural beliefs and practices.

These women's words sum up the cultural and developmental issues which influence the health status of women and children in Samoa, and clearly express the dilemma caused by a culture confronted with change.

4.2 The Traditional System

Samoa has tenaciously retained many of its traditional ways and practices and those of significance to maternal and child health are related to the traditional family structure, the land tenure system, and traditional medical practices and beliefs.

4.2.1 The Family or "Aiga"

The aiga (extended family) composed of several nuclear families is the traditional system in which the matai (head of the family) cares and provides for the welfare of family members.

It is essential to understand the traditional village and family social situation to plan and implement development. While some aspects of the traditonal Samoan social system limit economic development, it must be acknowledged that it has some virtues as the economic, social and political activities of the Samoan people are firmly rooted in the aiga and matai system. Within this, care is provided for the young, the old and sick, handicapped and the unemployed. There are provisions also for social services, through the church and other community activities.

4.2.2 Land tenure and distribution of food

Under the leadership of the matai, related persons pool their land, labour and other resources for subsistence cultivation of crops and raising of livestock for consumption, sale or export.

The aiga does not own the land, but holds a right to land use. It cannot be sold, though it can be leased. The insecurity of land use which affects individual families of the aiga is cited by some as one of the reasons for slow development. Thus the aiga - village farm families - hold 80% of Western Samoa's land resources and constitute nearly 70% of the labour resources.

While there is no shortage of food in Samoa, there is a problem of unequal distribution of food, not only between villages and families, but also within families. Food especially pigs, chickens and fish (in huge quantities) are highly valued and are an essential component for ceremonial exchanges of gifts. Traditionally, the matai and the village pastors receive the best and the most, with wives of untitled men and children picking at what is left over!

It is indeed ironic that infants and yound children are faced with a risk of undernourishment and even malnutrition while adults are almost always obese and consequently many suffer from diabetes, gout and hypertension.

Throughout our history, the nutrition and well-being of our people has been closely linked with the production and utilisation of indigenous crops. However, to feed an expanding population adequately, the local Department of Agriculture and the University of the South Pacific, School of Agriculture are researching new ways and methods of increasing food production, with emphasis on traditional crops.

4.2.3 Traditional Medicine and Traditional beliefs and practices relative to health

Well before the arrival of scientific medicine, the Samoans had a traditional health care system which included massaging to particular parts of the body, medicines made from leaves, stems and roots of certain plants, meditation with supernatural spirits and personal counselling more particularly by traditional healers (taulasea). Today, traditional medicine still plays an important role in rural communities where Western health care is not so readily available.

The traditional midwife has always held a special place in Samoan society. She is known as a "tufuga" which ranks her amongst those with special talents in the community. Consequently, her influence in family health is quite considerable.

The practice and skills of these traditional health practitioners has and is being studied, but not by Samoans. Unfortunately, the findings of these studies are not available to us at this time.

Hygienic and sanitary practices were ingrained in some of the cultural practices independent of the notion and the rationale of scientific medicine. Those practices are reflected in ceremonial occasions and can be observed in people's usual daily chores in the villages. Bathing for instance is a norm as mothers and children spend most of their time in the rivers and fresh water pools washing clothes, making tapa or simply gathering stones for their fale (house). The calling of the conch shell in the early part of the evening indicates the time for bathing and cleaning up before prayers and the evening meal.

Our traditional practices that promote good health of women and children are the special diet and care given to pregnant and lactating women and young infants, the encouragement of breastfeeding and the separation of the post-natal mother from her husband ("solifailele") until the infant and mother are well and strong. This practice of solifailele also helps to reduce the chance of early pregnancy.

It is inevitable that many of these good beliefs and practices are changing mainly because of an increasing trend towards individualistic achievements rather than promoting and sustaining the collective interests of the aiga and the village.

4.3 The Status of Women and Children

The status of women in modern Samoa is extremely complex and cannot be adequately described in one short paragraph. It is a well-known and well-documented fact that in old Samoa, the women enjoyed equal though ambivalent status with their menfolk. The only person at any time in history to hold all four paramount and kingly titles for the whole of Samoa was a woman - "Salamasina" - who lived somewhere in the fifteenth century. Throughout our history there are many other examples of women demonstrating this equal partnership with men in the traditional system.

Today that status and special place women as sisters and daughters once held in society has changed somewhat. The arrival of the missionaries and early colonialists with their so-called Christian and European beliefs and prejudices almost completely reversed the roles and status of women in Samoa. Penelope Schoffel has studied and brilliantly describes in her doctoral thesis titled "A Study of Gender, Status and Power in Western Samoa", (1979) the dynamics of this change.

In a tiny nutshell the high status of "sisters" and "daughters" which accorded females importance, dignity and esteem has been lowered, while the status of "wives" (except for wives of untitled men) has been elevated. Thus while the status of "sisters" and "daughters" was and still is legitimate, the status of "wives" is derived and conditional. It is fortunate however, that highly educated and talented women are recognised and can achieve high status. A number of these women have chiefly titles and are therefore entitled to sit with other matais in the village council or fono. Therefore today, women must be exceptional to an extent before they may enjoy high status or have the privilege to be part of the decision-making or policy making process for family or national development.

The changes over time on the status of children does not appear to be as profound. Traditionally the small child is given much love, care and attention, mostly from the older siblings, which could be either sister of brother. Since schools were introduced there were no longer so many older siblings to mind the younger ones with the result that grandparents or aunts had to be found to help out. Similarly as described by the grandmother in an earlier section, problems also arise when parents leave the village to earn more money elsewhere. These situations usually lead to adoption occasionally resulting in child neglect.

4.4 Community Participation and Women's Health Committees

The level of voluntary contribution and support by the various village groups to general development or to specific projects is recognised and noted by many international agencies.

There are traditional groupings of young untitled men of the village (aumaga), the sisters and daughters of the village (aualuma) as well as the Women's Committees, Education Committee and others.

4.4.1 Voluntary contribution

Samoan communities because of its unique social organisation, are noted for the very high contributions in various ways to the development of its own aiga (family), to the village and to the nation. It has been estimated that the savings to Government through the various communal activities, e.g. building district hospitals, health centres and staff living quarters, building village schools and churches etc., is in the region of thousands of tala (dollars) annually.

Furthermore when Government seeks voluntary assistance for its various village developmental activities there is usually a very positive response. In 1976 the Chief, Public Health Division, began a project to train young women as volunteer health aids to the District Health Service. Over 100 were trained by the district health staff. By 1980 only 25 remained. The enthusiasm of these young women gradually declined due largely to inadequate planning of the project, and poor definition of their tasks and their relationship with other formally trained staff. The young women were also given a number of unattained promises. Future volunteer projects will have to be designed with these mistakes in mind, but it is our belief that there is a real potential for greater utilisation of voluntary community involvement and assistance.

4.4.2 Women's Health Committees

What began in the 1920's as purely health oriented village women's organisation has now evolved into an organisation with very significant involvement in areas such as commercial agriculture, animal husbandry and handicraft manufacture. The membership is derived from the child-bearing women of the village but usually includes the widows, and older more highly respected women of the village, whether previously married or not.

For various reasons some women may be expelled or chose not to belong to the village health committee. This is seen as a real hindrance to providing a comprehensive health care service to these women and their families. The Health Department gives high priority to finding solutions to this problem.

Every village in Samoa has one or more women's committees and it is the members who form the backbone of the Rural Health Service. For it is these women, through their committees that arrange the village maternal and child health clinics, who build hospitals and health centres, provide caretaker services for these facilities, feed district doctors and nurses and help arrange village health campaigns. Village sanitation and beautification schemes are also heavily dependent on the initiative and support of the women's committees. Such activities have direct or indirect influence on the health status of the community and some Women's Committees have even started school lunch programmes.

4.5 Foreign Aid

Foreign aid has played a large part in the country's development effort especially in improving its infrastructure, health and other services, both directly and indirectly. In particular, food aid has made a considerable impact in improving the MCH situation in Western Samoa. A noted project amongst others, in this case is the World Food Programme Assistance for Nutrition Improvement of Vulnerable Groups which started in 1976. This involves distribution of dried skim milk powder to nursing and pregnant mothers and the needy pre-school children throughout Western Samoa. Even distribution of food aid as such is ensured with the assistance of the helpful and efficient women's committees and other social institutions. Other food aids such as canned fish is a cheap and easy way to get the necessary protein component of the basic diet.

4.6 Other Contributing Factors

A compounding factor is net-outmigration. Over the past period of years New Zealand has absorbed the largest share of migrants seeking employment. This has not only relieved the home country of population pressures but has also reaped the fruits of migration through the receiving of remittances. Remittances have contributed considerably to family welfare and life in the villages through improved housing, education, production and consumption and communal infrastructure such as churches, schools, electric plants and water schemes. For some families this is a major source of income. In 1979 it reached a level of seven million tala which helped ease the balance of payment problems. Too much reliance on remittances can be dangerous and may cause severe repercussions in the future as New Zealand is now tightening its immigration policies and there is difficulty also in migrating to

American Samoa and from there to the United States. Despite this, it is certain that remittances play a significant role in the standard of living in Samoan households and thus for maternal child care and health.

5. INTERSECTORAL HEALTH RELATED ACTIVITIES OR PROJECTS

A number of inter-related and intersectoral projects have directly contributed to improving the status of health of women and children in Samoa. Others, although such effects may not be immediately evident, do nevertheless have potential for strong positive effects sometime in the future.

5.1 Rural Development

The subsistance oriented village agricultural sector dominates Samoa's economic structure and involves two thirds of her labour force. It therefore deserves special attention in its development planning efforts in view of a growing population against a fixed resource base. Hence the formulation of a Rural Development Programme (RDP), an integral part of the Third Five Year Plan (1975-1979) and continuing through the Fourth Five Year Plan (1980-1984).

The RDP has two major objectives, stimulate village agricultural production and to foster a system of "planning from below". In Samoa, the second feature is probably a far more important factor. It takes advantage of the traditional form of local government found in Samoa -the village council of chiefs and orators as well as other existing social institutions such as the women's committees, youth groups and the aumaga or untitled men who carry out the will of the fono or village council. A Pulenuu who holds a chiefly nu'u-title is elected by the fono or becomes the village liaising agent with government.

The programme is administrated by a Rural Development Section of the Prime Mininster's Department and is a high government priority which demonstrates its commitment to meet the basic needs of the villages. From the outset there has been a strong support for an integrated approach. Firstly, to assist villages to plan for development in an intersectional way, but it also requires working toward a cooperative effort among the Government Departments, supporting villages' planning and implementation activities. Government or related services involved include the Department of Agriculture, especially its Advisory and Extension Division, field personnel of the Development Bank, the Departments of Health, Education and Public Works, field representatives of the Agricultural Store and the US Peace Corps, also Lands and Survey as needed.

A recent economic evaluation of the RDP showed that fishery projects, poultry farms, plantation shelters and development and water provision facilities and vegetable projects are all of economic benefit to the village as a whole. However, one only has to go to the market-place to witness the relatively abundant local produce such as taro and banana at low prices compared to say five years ago. A social evaluation of factors and influence of RDP on village life has not been carried out as yet, but this will be useful for future alternatives.

The most succesful village projects have been carried out by women. Considering the already organised strength of rural women in Samoa, it would not be possible to implement RDP especially when directed to the poorer sectors, without the support of women's groups. Their projects include poultry, cattle and vegetable raising projects, handicrafts, thatch and blind production, sale of marine products, fruits, copra and and various other enterprises. Villages that have been quick off the mark in taking advantage of assistance under RDP have been the better off villages as they are better organised,more commercially minded, enjoy good access to the town centre and have more (and accessible) land to develop. Consideration might be given to ways of stimulating the poorer villages.

The role of the RDP in villages which have implemented projects has certainly proven useful not only in increasing village agricultural production but has also increased community participation.

The majority of the activities of the Department of Agriculture are directed towards the provision of services for the village sector, both in relation to crops for export and crops and livestock for domestic consumption. It works closely with the RDP. Village access roads have undoubtedly assisted the movement of produce from more distant gardens and have facilitated the expansion of cultivated areas. Hence in the process rural producers and families are helped towards obtaining a fairer share of the fruits of development.

5.2 Income generating Projects for Women

Closely related to and often as an integral part of the RDP are the various income generating and village development projects organised by women. Most of the projects are begun through the initiative and drive of the women themselves, and others result from the advisory activities of the Women's Advisory Committee.

Appreciating the significant, though largely unrecognised role of women in social and economic development, the Government of Western Samoa formed in 1979 an Advisory Committee for Women with direct access and being responsible to the

Prime Minister. Contrary to the wishes of a number of women the members were personally selected by the Prime Minister to serve a term of three years. Attempts by this Committee therefore to function as an efficient coordinating and unifying body of the many women's organisation existing in Samoa, have largely been unsuccessful.

It has however been fairly successful in stimulating, promoting and assisting in the various activities for generating income more particularly in the handicraft industry. Workshops have also been organised aimed at teaching skills for self and family life improvement, home economics, improving family health etc. The appropriate officials from governmental and non-governmental sectors have assisted in these workshops.

5.3 Home Economics through the Department of Agriculture

In 1979 the Department of Agriculture set-up a Home Economics Unit under its Agricultural Extension Programme. This Unit consist of two highly skilled and dynamic women who traval around the islands teaching rural and urban women the principle of better family life, through budgeting, planning of nutritious and economical family meals and applying simple and appropriate technology for village living. The emphasis is on more efficient utilisation of local and readily available low-cost resources.

5.4 The Contribution of Church to health

Almost every Samoan professes affiliation or strong adherence to one of the several Christian churches operating in Samoa. Of these, the Seventh Day Adventist and the Church of Jesus Christ of Latter Day Saints have been most outstanding in their teaching and promotion of good health and sound health practices.

It is impossible to show what effects this may have on the health of their church members but we believe that these people are amongst the healthiest in Samoa.

The missions are always interested and supportive of health campaigns and it is not surprising therefore that the Health Department recognises their leaders and takes every opportunity to involve and consult them where appropriate.

5.5 Education through the formal and non-formal sectors

The education of a Samoan child starts very early with all the family members playing a part - which sometimes can be conflicting.

Almost right from the beginning of the conversion of Samoans to christianity in the 1830's, the churches have been involved with training and education of their adherents and their children. The pastors schools account for the very high literacy level of Samoan men and women - a level in the region of 98%.

Formal pre-school education is also provided by the Pre-School Association through its centres scattered throughout Samoa. This rapidly expanding association involves parents (usually mothers) and their children who therefore learn together in the process. By closely working and involving the mothers, there is the opportunity for adult education and the Pre-school Association has developed extensive plans for achieving this objective.

Although going to school is not compulsory, nor is it free or even inexpensive, the acquisition of knowledge, especially the palagi (European) knowledge is highly valued for it is regarded as a passport to well-paid jobs. From analysing the figures contained in the 1976 Census report, 78% of the population of children aged 5-19 years were enrolled at school. Of this 51.2% were males and 48.8% were females -an extremely encouraging proportion. Almost every child starts school at 5 1/2 years but begin dropping out after 5-6 years of schooling. Reasons for dropping out include low family income, being needed to help with family chores or personal preference.

Recognising that perhaps 90% of the school population will never leave Samoa, the Department of Education has placed an emphasis or a bias for technical courses called "provocational". It aims at giving some information and understanding of the basic technological skills that are already in existence in Western Samoa e.g. basic understanding of electricity, carpentry, plumbing, marketing, credit, house-keeping, budgeting, food nutrition and so on. The bias is regarded as useful and can even be introduced at the primary level, as those who do not go beyond junior high school level would return to the villages having acquired some knowledge as well as some practical skills which they can usefully apply in their daily work.

In Samoa, there is wide community involvement in its education system. The villages usually construct and maintain their own primary and Junior High Schools and the churches make a significant contribution towards pre-school right through to secondary education, thus saving government thousands of tala. All these factors have played a role in raising the level of education within the community to what it is now and is an important contributing factor to the level of maternal and child health.

5.6 Health Education

It is surprising to us that Western Samoa has only very recently established a Health Education Section within the Department of Health. Previously the District Nurses were required to give health talks during their meetings and clinics with the Women's Committees, but they received little if any training for this.

The Department of Education also includes basic hygiene in the curriculum for primers but health teaching for older children is most inadequate and urgently needs review to include such subjects as family life education and problems arising from uncontrolled population growth.

The potential and real effect of the mass media as agents of change is also realised. Apia boasts of eight weekly news-papers, at least one for every day of the week, not including periodic government and church newspapers.

The possession of a radio is a must for most Samoan families. A survey of household living conditions in 1971-1972 found that 80% of rural households have radio which, given the communal nature of village life, means virtually 100% access. The Broadcasting Department fulfils an important role being the principal medium for news and educational programmes, advertising and personal communications (many telegrams being delivered by radio) and also Government Information. It is the only radio station in Western Samoa. Forty-five per cent of the population receive a poor signal and projects are now underway in setting up new transmitting stations. The Broadcasting service works closely with Government departments and voluntary organisation in the compilation of their programmes. A favourite which attracts a wide range of listeners is a Women's Development Programme featuring advice to women on a variety of topics including child care, nutrition, recipes using local ingredients, and interviews with noted women. Development spots including family planning announcements in conjunction with the Family Welfare Services of the Health Department are inter-spaced with music and drama. Another important attraction of listening to the radio is the nightly broadcasts of money-order recipients announcing the names and villages of the recipients who then travel to the nearest Post Office to pick up their money-orders.

The high level of literacy, the high development and popularity of the mass media and the thirst of knowledge are all important factors which will be more fully utilised and developed by the new Health Education Section.

6. PRIORITIES AND PLANS FOR MCH

In our efforts to provide a comprehensive health care service to the majority of the population, it is inevitable that certain vulnerable groups will be deprived to some extent. These groups will include non-Women's Committee Members, low income families especially those living in the Apia urban area, displaced families through urbanisation or moving inland to cultivate land and the physically and mentally disabled. The Family Welfare Section (FWS) of the Health Department has defined high risk factors for women and children but there have been some reluctance by some of the staff to adopt the high-risk approach. This is because they feel they are obliged to give the same amount of time and attention to everyone - even if those persons are healthy and well.

Nevertheless, we believe that the priorities or targets for MCH during the next 10 years are:

(a) to lower the birth rate to less than 30/100 population

(b) to lower the incidence of early childhood malnutrition especially in rural Upolu and in the Apia urban are;

(c) to provide non-Women's Committee members with adequate MCH care and to encourage them to belong to a Women's Committee;

(d) to further promote the spirit of voluntary effort in order to stimulate and train selected members of the community to take more responsibility for the health of their children, families, for themselves and other village members; and

(e) to significantly improve the efficiency and accuracy of the vital registration system as well as the whole health information system, in order to better evaluate our activities and plan for future needs.

To meet these priorities, new projects and activities have begun or are being proposed.

6.1 <u>The Population Policy and FP targets</u>

The Fourth Five Year Development Plan 1980-1984 includes a Population Policy, which recognises the urgent need for population control and outlines an intersectoral approach to slow down the currently high growth rate.

The policy emphasises the need to motivate and to educate men, and the FWS has outlined such a programme.

A FP campaign is to be carried out late in 1981 and the planning and execution of this campaign will closely involve other sectors of government and NGO's especially the churches. How to overcome religious and cultural attitudes somewhat resistant to educating young people about human reproduction and responsible parenthood is a long standing challenge.

6.2 Activities for improved nutrition

6.2.1 Food and Nutrition Policy

As a result of a highly successful WHO sponsored seminar on Nutrition held in Apia in November 1980 a Food and Nutrition Policy was drafted. This document needs to be discussed and accepted by Cabinet before any real changes can be expected. The seminar included many representatives from relevant government departments, from the commercial sector, from NGO's including the churches, and it generated a lot of interest and discussion between the participants.

6.2.2 Maternity Protection

A small sub-committee of the Occupational Health Committe is at present preparing a report on the need for and estimated costs of a Maternity Protection scheme. Two of the authors of this paper are members of this sub-committee. The provision of adequate maternity protection will not only protect the health and rights of working women but also the nutritional status and health of their new borns.

6.2.3 Better Infant Feeding Campaign

This campaign is soon to start and is aimed particularly at members who do not breastfeed or who wean too soon. It is planned to be carried out over a six month period and goals and strategies have been worked out. A Planning Committee representing the mass media, the Education and Health Department is responsible.

6.2.4 Control of Diarrhoel Disease of early childhood

Although no definite project is planned for the immediate future, we appreciate that the control of diarrhoel diseases need attention. The very close interaction with malnutrition is recognised but environmental measures such as improved excreta disposal, adequate uncontaminated water supplies are perhaps more important at present.

Rehydration salts are available but they have not been properly distributed nor have the staff or public been fully instructed on their proper use.

6.3 Increase Community Participation

It is appreciated that Samoa already has a high level of voluntary and community assistance to health and other developmental programmes - perhaps higher than in many other developing countries. This is possible because of the nature of our culture and form of social organisation and because we are a relatively small country. Nevertheless we believe that we can further stimulate communities, not to build more district hospitals or health centres but to take more responsibilities for their own health, to assist the district nurses to monitor certain conditions and to report vital events in the village.

Plans are being prepared for achieving these objectives which will be executed by the Family Welfare and Health Education Sections, with the involvement of the Women's Advisory Committee and Pre-School Association.

It is also hoped that a training programme for new village Health Workers and TBA's will be started sometime in 1982.

6.4 Improved Health Information and Vital Registration System

6.4.1 Reporting and Recording of MCH Activities

This is being revised and will soon be put on trial. Some radical changes have been made, but if the system is succesful it will be adopted nationally next year.

A home-based Child Health Record will also be put on trial at the same time, and it is our hope that in a few years this record will be regarded as a passport for school entry, as the birth certificate is today.

6.4.2 Vital Registration

The Department of Health is currently collaborating with the Department of Statistics and the Pulenu'u (village mayors) in an attempt to improve the registration of births and deaths. Because of the special relationship between the District Nurse (DN) and the village under her care, the DN is increasingly being asked to act as the eyes and ears of important village events. Selected members of the Women's Committees are also envisaged as assisting in this important activity.

7. SUMMARY AND CONCLUSION

Western Samoa is ranked amongst the least developed nations of the world. This does hurt our national pride, but we know that the indicators on which such ranking is based do not and cannot explain the relative abundance of food, the absence of visible suffering from disease, improved village housing, and the widespread distribution of village schools, health centres and consumer goods. These attributes are a result of a number of inter-related socio-economic factors, the social organisations, institutions and practices which exist in Samoa as well as government's efforts through its departmental services and developmental programmes to provide a solid basis for self-sustained economic growth and improvements in the quality of life. The interaction of these factors are described, particularly as they relate to or influence the health status of women and children in Samoa.

But unless Samoa is able to significantly lower the growth of population and improve its export earnings, the rising expectation of the people will lead to major problems. Furthermore it must also be stated that deliberate changes and plans, all too often move at a snail's place. The frustrations of trying to introduce or implement new projects often discourage and drive away many of our best trained and skilled persons. To succeed and remain effective one needs to have incredible patience, a good sense of humour, an intimate knowledge and understanding of the "faa-Samoa" (the Samoan way) and a deep love and pride of the country. Such qualities are not easy to find, but with the combined efforts of a number of key persons in different sectors of the community, the future for women and children in Samoa is bright.

8. ACKNOWLEDGEMENTS

We wish to express our thanks to the many people who so kindly gave us their time to talk to us and share with us their knowledge and experience.

9. BIBLIOGRAPHY

Brazil H., Factors in Early Childhood Malnutrition in Western Samoa (mimeograph). Health Department, Apia, 1979.

Department of Health, (1980), Health Statistics for Western Samoa 1979, Government of Western Samoa, Apia, 1980.

Department of Health, (1980), Annual Report of the Health Department 1979, Government of Western Samoa, Apia, 1980.

Department of Health, (1981), Annual Report of the Family Welfare Section 1980 (mimeograph) Apia, 1981.

Department of Economic Development, (1976), Western Samoa's Third Five Year Development Plan 1976-1979, Government of Western Samoa, Apia, 1980.

Department of Economic Development, (1980), Western Samoa's Five Year Development Plan 1980-1984. Vol. 1. Government of Western Samoa, Apia, January, 1980.

Department of Statistics, (1980), Annual Statistical Abstracts 1979, Government of Western Samoa, Apia, 1980.

Department of Statistics, (1979), Census of Population and Housing 1976, Analytical Report vol. 2, Government of Western Samoa, Apia.

Jansen A.A.J., (1977), Malnutrition and Child Feeding Practices in Western Samoa, Environmental Child Health. December, 1977, 293-306.

Leung Wai S.G., (1975), Problems of Transition in a Dual Economy - The case of Western Samoa. Sub-thesis for a Masters in Agricultural Development Economics. Australian National University, Canberra 1975.

Schoeffel P., (1979), A study of Gender, Status and Power in Western Samoa. A doctoral thesis for the Australian National University; Canberra, Australia.

Quested C., Breastfeeding and Artificial Feeding Practices in Western Samoa (mimeograph), Health Department, Apia, 1978.

Wood C., Gans L.P., (1981), Haemobological status of Reproductive Women in Western Samoa. An Analysis of Biometric Data. Human Biology, May 1981, Vol.53, No.2, pp 269-279.

Zimmert P. et al, (1980), Blood Pressure Studies in Rural and Urban Western Samoa. The Medical Journal of Australia 1980, 2 : 202-205.

ANNEXE

A. ESTIMATED DEMOGRAPHIC AND OTHER CHARACTERISTICS OF WESTERN SAMOA - 1979

Population	..	160,000
Crude birth rate	..	35/1000 population
Crude death rate	..	7.5/1000 "
Actual growth rate (%)	..	1.71
Total fertility rate	..	6.7
% of population under 15 yrs.	..	46.9
Infant mortality rate	..	36/1000 live births
Life expectancy at birth	..	60 yrs for males 63 yrs for females
Literacy rate	..	98%
Net emigration as % of population	..	1.25

Sources: A variety of Government publications.

B. OTHER INDICATORS OR MATERNAL AND CHILD HEALTH - 1980

1. Child Health

Percent of infants (011 mths) with Child Health records	..	81.4%
Percent of preschoolers (14 yrs) with Child Health records	..	72.6%
Percent of children with completed immunisation	..	43.8%
* Percent of children 0-3 yrs with malnutrition	..	19.5%
** Average age of Infants at weaning	..	7.3 months

2. Maternal Health

Average percentage of pregnant women attending antenatal clinic	..	80%
Average gestational age of foetus at first visit	..	25 weeks
Mean blood haemoglobin concentration during pregnancy	..	10.8-11.4 gs/100 mls
Percent of births attended by TBA's	..	40-50%
*** Percent of women 15-49 yrs currently using a family planning method	..	15%

Sources: Report of the Evaluation Study of the MCH/FP Project Health Department (not published)

* Brazill H. 1980
** Quested C. 1979
*** Health Department - Result of Current User Survey - September 1980 (not published)

CHAPTER SEVEN

THE STATES OF DEVELOPMENTAL HEALTH IN FOUR CARIBBEAN ISLANDS: APPROACHING THE FORTUNES OF INFANT HEALTH AND WELFARE *

1. INITIAL OBSERVATIONS

In the early 1970s, I undertook to study empirically the state of development at the international level (1). In this study, I conceived development and underdevelopment rather unfashionably as the properties of the world's international system and not those of any particular part of it; and I approached the subject in the then familiar context of bridging the development gap between the centre and the periphery of the world-system.

I used certain measures to estimate the extent to which the developmental gap could be said to have narrowed between 1960 and 1970 on eight developmental value-indicators. Included in the measures were (2): the Concordance Level (Spearman's rank-order correlation coefficient, Rho);

*Paper prepared by Herb Addo, University of West Indies, Trinidad.

The Systems Inequality Measure (SIM); four measures derived from Lorenz Curves, namely the Gini Index, the Equal Share Coefficient, the Ratio of Discrimination, and the location of the Dynamic Middle of Lorenz Curves (3). Among the value-indicators employed were: GNP *per capita*; Energy Consumption *per capita* (4); Combined Adjusted Primary and Secondary School Enrollment Ratio; Number of Students in Third Level Education *per* 100,000 Population; Circulation of Daily and Non-Daily Newspaper *per* 1,000 Population; Calories *per* Day *per* Inhabitant; Population *per* Physician; and Infant Mortality Rates.

After complex manipulation of the enormous data gathered on all independent nations in the world, I came to the worrisome conclusion that not much could be said to have changed developmentally between the centre and the periphery during the period 1960-1970. Even more distressing was the finding that a study of the African particularity within the developmental *problématique* showed that during the decade, when much was said on Africa and much appeared to have been done in and for Africa developmentallly, not much difference showed for African nations on the constructed developmental indices.

In the course of this exercise, I noticed that for some countries there appeared to be the happy situation where low GNP *per capita* went along with "high scores" on other value-indicators. Most interestingly these value-indicators included IMR. The Caribbean nations for which I had data, notable Trinidad and Barbados, fell in this category of nations.

The natural question that agitated my mind then was: why? My unreflected response to this teasing question was that, not unlike the animals on "the farm", all Third World countries were poor but some were clearly poorer than others.

I have been living in the Caribbean since March 1973 (5). During this more than eight-year period, I have silently but reflectively observed that unlike the children in most parts of Africa that I know (in particular Ghana my native country), the children in the Caribbean seem to be in "visible" good health. What was even more interesting to me was that, from my casual observation, I noticed that visible good health did not appear to be visibly related to socio-economic status of parents, their marital status, or the distance of their locations from the centre of regions and countries where health and other services have the unfortunate habit of concentrating. This is not to say that there are no child health and welfare problems in the Caribbean. It is to say that perhaps they are not as bad as one would expect given our unsatisfactory conception of development, because of its excessive economistic and its large Eurocentric imitative endowment (6).

2. THE RESEARCH QUESTION: ITS MEANING

If, therefore, the question is why child health and welfare in the Caribbean does not fit a conventional mode of expectation, then, for conceptutal and analytical purposes, we must ask, to be sure of what answers we are seeking: what really is the question?

My appreciation of the matter is that the project is not asking anything of child health and welfare as such. It seeks only to ascertain the fortunes of child health and welfare. The real question is addressed to the socioeconomic aspects and/or the non-health variables which affect child health and welfare.

Approached this way, we know immediately that the matter we are dealing with is the relationship(s) between socioeconomic variables and the fortunes of child health and welfare. Our dependent variable is child health and welfare and our independent variable is a cluster of socioeconomic varibales. Once we approach the matter this way, we know when we have a problem and when we don't. By this I mean that if the developmental meaning we accord the cluster of socioeconomic variables, that is their developmental health, squares with the particular fortunes of child health and welfare in the context of our conventional conception of development, then we do not have any problem (7). We have a problem which demands answers to the question why only if in the context of our conventional conception of development, we perceive some disparity between the independent and the dependent variables. It is only when we encounter such a disparity that we ask: why is the Caribbean different in this regard from other developmentally comparable regions within the Third World.

Attempting to answer this question will take us back not to the fortunes of child health and welfare, but back to our very conventional conception of development and its economistic and Eurocentric endowments. We will then have to ask ourselves whether development should continue to mean the development of things to facilitate the accumulation of capital, which then reflects, intentionally or unintentionally, in many social forms including good fortunes for child health and welfare; whether we are to conceive development in terms of the enhancing human dignity which therefore implies good fortunes for child health and welfare.

What I am suggesting here then is that this research could lead to many fundamental implications. We may have to redefine our very conception of "poverty situation", but we cannot escape confronting what I have called elsewhere the peculiarity of the Caribbean plight within the generalized plight of the periphery of the world-system.

To even understand a deceptively limited matter as the state of IMRs of four Caribbean Islands, demands some understanding of why the Caribbean as part of the periphery is very much different from it. We cannot understand vital difference outside the crucial historical terms of how and why history, as contemporary presence of the past, makes it so.

We cannot answer the question as to whether the fortunes of child health and welfare in the Caribbean is the result of deliberate policy of intersectoral action or a fortuitous spin-off from sectorial effect, without reference to the peculiar identity of the Caribbean as it has been shaped by world-history to date.

One cannot write meaningfully about the Caribbean without referring to the difficulties involved in defining what constitutes the Caribbean area. Neither can one write meaningfully in 1980 about the historic plight of the area and its transformational destiny without respecting the fact that the Caribbean is not just a part of the capitalist world-system but the oldest part of the periphery of the world-economy. I shall argue that the Caribbean is unique within the periphery and, for this reason, the Caribbean plight assumes a peculiarity of its own within the generalized plight of the periphery. I shall argue further that because of this peculiarity the Caribbean probably bears a special responsibility for the transformational destiny of the capitalist world-system as a whole.

The elements which constitute the Caribbean plight at this phase of the world-system can be represented by the small size of the states and the economies in the Caribbean, and the long history of this area's participation in the world-economy. The Caribbean is small, and if this smallness is taken together with the long participation in world-history, it points to the peculiarity of the Caribbean area within the group of peripheral states. The peculiarity is precisely the depth and the breadth of the penetration of the Caribbean area by dominant capital (8).

When my argument comes to be fully elaborated it will indicate that, as world-history moves on, the Caribbean shows other peripheral states and societies the image of their own future. This could mean many things that are "bad" and therefore undesirable, but it could also mean better child health and welfare even in a conventionally defined "poverty situation".

From the above, we are in a much better position to appreciate the meanings of the analytical-methodological questions which we must put, if we are to pursue the research curiosity as presented above. The following are some of the questions we must pose, if we are to proceed:

1. Is any perceived disparity due to a difference in health culture which can be explained in terms of a different mix between modern and traditional Caribbean medicines, conceptions of health, and the very conception of the child?

2. Is this difference to be explained in terms of deliberate policy of government, which in turns is to be explained in terms of the closer colonial links which existed

between the Caribbean Islands and their metropoles; in fact, in the physical presence in large numbers of the colonialists in the Islands and the enforced, even if discriminatory, close contact between the people and the colonialists?

3. Is this, then, a beneficial legacy of the painful colonial experience, which in the end translates into good prenatal, neonatal, and other child care good fortunes such as the innoculation culture?

4. Or is it due to the accessibility and good maintenance of health clinics, even in situations where health services are in utter disarray?

5. Is the accessibility to be explained in terms of, and among other things, the comparative (9) small size of these Islands?

6. Is this further assisted by reasonably and comparatively good road system, which reduce, if not remove, the urban-rural distance, thus making prenatal, natal and postnatal cares almost routine and hence culturally a norm?

A careful reading of this proposal up to this point will inidicate that these questions above are not arbitrary. The method is really in the questions, the relationships between them, and their overall relevance to the real question as formulated above, in early parts of this section.

What method shall we use then to answer this real question?

3. METHODOLOGY

I shall say two things on this. First, not until one formulates a research question properly, it is futile to exert thought on the methods for pursuing the question. Second, once a question has been formulated properly, the methods for its pursuit, within the limits of an existing epistemology, comes naturally. Given the formulation of our question, it is clear to see that all methods are relevant, but none of them is indispensable. This means that, while all known methods can be used, it is the formulation of the main question that leads to the logical methods in a given epistemology. We therefore have all the traditional methods available for the study of the subject to choose from.

To make our choice of methods clear, we must specify our methodology, that is we must state why we approach the subject the way we do. This research will be conducted in the belief that important social issues of the kind that our topic is, must always be approached via the simplest methodologies. Therefore, even though the methodology for studying human development of which our topic is a part, has undergone tremendous changes over the last decade, all of which changes cannot be considered laudatory, I shall stick as much as possible to a mix of statistical methods which are suitable for enlightening felt and observed qualitative situations.

The methodology will consist of combing existing literature for reasons why the initial observations should or should not be so (10). In the course of this exercise, there may be reasons to revise the initial observations. Where statistics and other hard avenues allow, I shall employ them not so much to explain as to describe the situation as clearly as they can.

I adopt this way of approaching the question because my interest at this phase of the project is not to measure anything as such, but to describe and perhaps explain a curious qualitative human situation: measurement takes second place in the commonsensical explanation of this curious qualitative human situation in a given historical context. My main methodological concern is to put my initial observations and intuitive explanations not to a complex validating statistical tests, but to describe them where possible by statistical light.

The four Islands that will be studied are Trinidad and Tobago, Barbados, Grenada and Antigua. These Islands are very different in their socio-demographic make-up. I shall omit the detailed description of the differences at the moment. Suffice it to say that the extent that these Islands differ among themselves and the extent that they are similar, because they are all Caribbean, should make for a rich pilot research project. Given the time span of the research and other things, it should be clear that we can only scratch the surface of this interesting project, but we must scratch it in such a way that we like to scratch further.

NOTES

(1) Herb Addo, "Trends and Patterns in African Participation in International Relations, 1960-1970: Toward a Theory of International Realtions", unpublished Ph.D. thesis, Department of Political Science, Carleton University, 1974.

(2) See Herb Addo "Trends and Patterns in Value-Inequality 1960-1970: An Empirical Study", Journal of Peace of Research. 1976, 13(1): 13-34.

(3) The "dynamic middle" is the name I gave the sensitive parts of the Lorenz Curves as regards the group of nations most likely to improve their situations on a value-indicator. I discuss this variant of path analysis which I devised in the reference in note 1 above, chapter 5. See also my "International Value-Inequality 1960-1970: Periphery Nations in the 'Dynamic Middle' of Lorenz Curves, "Caribbean Yearbook of International Relations, 1975, pp. 158-187.

(4) The use of this indicator clearly shows the limits of our developmental thinking in the early 1970s. This was, of course, before Limits to Growth and OPEC alerted us all.

(5) I lived nearly two and half years in Guyana from 1973, I have been living in Trinidad since 1975, and I have visited and observed the other Islands in the region rather extensively.

(6) For what I mean by Eurocentric and imitative conception of development see my manuscript on "World-System Critique of Eurocentric Conception of Imperialism", 1981, especially chapter 1. See also my "Globale Ökonomie und eurozentrische Theorie: Eine Kritiktraditionelle Imperialismustheorie", in Foker Frobel et al. (ed.), Krisen in der Kapitalistischen Weltökonomie. Hamburg: Rowohlt, 1981, pp.194-235; as well as my "Strategic Aspects of the New International Economic Order's Developmental Potential", forthcoming in George Aseniero (ed.), Development.

(7) See the references in note 6 above. We would then have merely confirmed the conventional wisdom that underdevelopment as we conceive it goes with and includes poor child health and welfare. The Caribbean is important in this project because it threatens to prove otherwise.

(8) See my "Peculiarity of the Caribbean Plight", HSDRGPID-24/UNUP-135, 1980 and my "Caribbean Prospects for the 1980s: The Plight and the Destiny", mimeo, December 1980.

(9) The concept small as it pertains to the size of states, that is the concept small-state, has been discussed at some length in my references in note 9 above. The comparative component of this complex concept refers to comparative attributive smallness of Caribbean states.

(10) Many such sources exist in the literature on the Caribbean. I shall omit detailed references. Rich statistical and other sources can be found in all the Islands' equivalent of statistical offices, even if in a somewhat confused form. In Trinidad, the Institute of Social and Economic Studies, UWI, has an impressive monograph series on aspects of this subject.

CHAPTER EIGHT

TIME & HEALTH/DEVELOPMENT
MCH IN ETHIOPIA*

FOREWARD**

There has been much concern lately about the inadequacies of measuring, monitoring and evaluating health and development and assessing costs and benefits. Some of the trouble has arisen from fuzzy definitions of both health and development themselves, but much is also due to the measuring rods used. We are suggesting that much more attention should be paid to time. Implicit in many analyses is that people in the third world have time on their hands, that they are idle or unemployed.

The following paper, applying a time budget analysis to Ethiopian materials show that this is an ethnocentric idea. In fact an unfortunate and unrecognized feature of western industrialization has been that many people, especially

* Paper prepared by Solomon Ayalew

** David Pitt, WHO/MCH/HQ

in developing countries, have now lost control over much of their own time without any very obvious benefits in goods or spare time. In many developing countries the effects of the introduction of cash cropping or wage labour etc. have been to make people work long hours, often in unpleasant situations, or inequitable social relationships, simply to live on the breadline, which takes much more time than, say, a living from traditional kinds of subsistence activity. Apart from the working hours themselves, there is the time of preparation (education) and relocation (migration). Even the 'spare time' produced by leisure, seasonality and unemployment may be mitigated by time lost in sickness.

Health services notably maternal and child health services, should have had a positive role in producing more time in the process of development. Preventing premature (notably child) mortality, extending expectancies of life all produce more time. Less time is lost when sick days can be reduced. But there are countervailing pressures. The long journeys some people have to make to clinics, the long waits for treatment and generally delays and blockages in communications, the relatively high costs of sometimes even essential drugs in some countries, the time lost from work or leisure because of ineffective medical services are all negative factors. The low costs of time in the developing world have been cited too as a reason for high fertility*.

There are several ways of involving time in the health/development measurement problematique. One is to include time in cost/benefit analyses. However here one cannot escape the problems associated with money (and its overlapping and

* Ho T.J. - 1974 - Time costs of child rearing in rural Philippines - Population & Development Review 5 (4) 643-62.

often confused) functions. An alternative may be time-budgeting, or more precisely a balance sheet of any activity, including MCH, of time lost and time gained, where alternative and more effective allocations of time become a prime concern of planning. Here emphasis is given not only to how people allocate (or are forced to allocate) their time. Finally it is not only the lineal increases or decreases in time that are important, but also the articulation of the introduced and indigenous time systems. For example health interventions may be as effective if they are timely, i.e. in relation to special times of risk or times of need of communities and individuals. This paper from Ethiopia argues powerfully for a closer and more careful analysis of time at the grass roots to improve MCH and to allow communities to achieve a self-reliant development appropriate to local conditions and aspirations.

1. MCH AND DEVELOPMENT IN ETHIOPIA*

The underdeveloped countries (UDC) may be classified on the basis of gross product per capita into low income countries with per capita income of US$ 300 and below, and middle income countries with a per capita income of + US$ 300 (1)(8). Ethiopia with a per capita income of about US$ 100 and which trails way behind most low income countries is in the UN classification of least developed countries.

One major cause and effect of least development is infant mortality and morbidity(9). The official infant mortality rate is estimated to be 155 per 1000 live births and the official child mortality to be 247 per 1000 live births or about 400 000 child deaths per year. Maternal mortality (9,11) is one of the highest in the world. Life expectancy is hardly 40 years.

*The author gratefully acknowledges the help of W. Almaz, T. Ayletch, G. Yoseph, B. Tewabetch, T. Meharia, G. Elias (Ethiopia) and Dr. G. Sterky and Dr. D.C. Pitt (WHO)

From a total number of 4 million malnourished children it is estimated that about 10% (or 400 000) are in a state of starvation (Marasmus) and 5% (200 000) manifest severe energy and protein deficiency (Kwashiorkor). The population of under-nourished children has an annual increase of about 200 000. The nutritional problem is aggravated in a form of localized famines which occur every year, whilst serious famines although occurring less frequently, have a more serious effect on a much larger population(2)(3)(4)(5). The most recent example is the 1973/74 famine of Wollo and Tigrai Regions which affected 2.6 million people, in which over 200 000 people died. Even in the ordinary times where famine is absent most of the children who receive treatment in the health establishment are underweight(6)(7). However if most infant mortality occurs amongst 20% of the population, even these deaths are preventable. In one study of patients in childrens' wards, where 14 out of a total of 104 died, it was observed that 10 deaths (71%) would have been avoided if the children had been brought to the hospital earlier(10)(11). Another study into the causes of maternal deaths showed that most of these could have been prevented if there had been a wide network of health services and if the smaller health units were organized to handle MCH problems(12).

Our argument here is that a major reason for MCH problems was that the health services failed to understand and to accommodate patterns of time use in the communities or on the periphery. This has resulted in relatively high IMRs in Ethiopia(13). Other countries which have mobilized their MCH services have drastically reduced infant mortality rate(14)(15) and we will argue this has important economic benefits and is a necessary prerequisite for agricultural development(16).

2. TIME BUDGET ALLOCATIONS IN RURAL COMMUNITIES

The meaning of budget in the financial sense is well known. Here we use budget concept in the same sense except that the resource under consideration is not finance but time measured in numbers of days. However, unlike a financial budget for which there are legal provisions and constraints a time budget is governed by customary laws. It is a societal norm that sick friends and neighbours have to be visited, funeral ceremonies, weddings and church holidays should be attended. People failing to comply with the set of the community's standards will face ostracism or even physical abuse.

That is why time allotments will ordinarily not change without very good reason. If contingencies arise, there may be a transfer of time. For example, if epidemics enter the region in the month of Tir, weddings may be deferred to the next year.

The following is an outline of the allocation of time resources in everyday activities in the community.

3. PRODUCTIVE LABOUR

Because of widespread mortality the population structure is deformed in the sense that the unproductive age group predominates over the productive age group. Agricultural tools and implements are very simple, consisting chiefly of a wooden plough with an iron wedge. Because of the low productivity of labour the execution of even limited activities takes a considerable time.

In table 1 the time budget allocation of the people of Tigrai for the year 1981 is shown. For the year 1981 112 days (31% of the year) are allocated for productive work. This pattern of time budget allocation appears to represent the regions of Gojjam, Gondar and part of the regions of Wollo and Showa, covering at least 40% of the total population of approximately 30 million people.

There are also indications that the maximum use of time available for productive work in Tigrai also reflects time use in other parts of the country. This may be observed from the fact that despite the sweeping land reform of 1975 which entitled every peasant household up to 10 hectares of land (and despite the availability of large expanses of unfarmed land) the increase of land under cultivation was negligible. This indicates that under existing conditions the nation has reached the full use of the time available for productive work (Table 2).

4. MORBIDITY AND MORTALITY

The impact of illness or death on time budgets of the community is apparent everywhere. The effect of illness with recurrent acute episodes which may occur at critical times such as planting and harvesting (e.g. malaria) creates a demand for additional labour supply or calls for a reallocation of time from other activities to productive labour time. When the problem is acute and temporary this may simply involve an increased work effort from other members of the family. However, debilitating diseases which impair active work for long periods require other solutions. One sure way of getting more labour is to produce more children.

Illness or death are social occasions where people congregate to mourn or to offer condolence and have serious implications on the time budget. During a period of mourning, immediate families suspend work for at least seven days while friends and distant relatives are expected to devote three full days of their time to be with the families of the deceased. This is in addition to keeping them company for about three hours of each day for a period of not less than 15 days. On average it is estimated that such activities account for 5% of the total budget (Table 1).

Each year there are approximately 300 infant deaths and at least 100 people congregate for around seven days to mourn each death. The total number of days lost is in the region of 2.1 millions per year or over 6000 man years. If we assume that mortality conditions are the tip of the iceberg of overall health conditions of the people in Ethiopia, the communities time burden will certainly be much greater. Some of the activities connected with mortality and morbidity coincide with holidays so that the estimate of 5% of the total time (Table 1) represents only a portion of the time lost.

5. REPRODUCTION

As we have seen, in order to obtain a reliable source of labour supply, many families try to have as many children as possible (Table 3).

In one survey, 46% of parents expressed their desire for a greater number of children to assist them in work and old age, thus indicating the short supply of labour. This response was given despite the belief that the areas are assumed from the outside to be densely populated.

For example the density of rural Dessie Zuria Awraja is 181.8 per sq. km as compared with 16.92 for rural Ethiopia and is the highest in the country(20). The remaining 56% of the families also want a large number of children. 25% appreciated God's beneficence, 22% simply appreciated children and 9% wanted to increase the number of relatives.

Childbirth is also a time consuming activity. Birth itself is a great occasion for celebration and extravagance as well as a cause for a break from work. To this should be added the time lost during pregnancy, for a mother's work output declines for approximately six months (before and after delivery)(17), requiring additional labour to assist in the house. The loss in time for the family increases dramatically if there is maternal mortality, the risk of which increases with each birth. The time associated with childbirth is estimated to be approximately 1% (again excluding times that coincide with holidays).

6. HOLIDAYS

Both national and religious holidays have a share of the time budget. In 1980 national holidays which number 13 (with only 7% of them falling on working days) (Table 4) are far less than non-governmental and non-official holidays.

For the Christians there is a church holiday every day of the month repeating throughout the 12 months of the year, although not all communities celebrate all holidays. Although the choice of holiday observance may differ from place to place, on the average orthodox-Christians in rural communities observe approximately 15 holidays every month (when Saturdays and Sundays are included). Even in Addis Ababa, the capital citiy, religious observance is as widespread. Religious holidays which may cost the rural population up to 46% of their time budget reflect mortality and morbidity and the hardships of life which people face. Widespread ill-health and poverty over which the individual community has no control, has led many to look at life with fatalistic resignation (18)(19).

7. POLITICAL PARTICIPATION

The 1974 Revolution which gave land to the peasants and called for new organization to defend their interests, resulted in new community activities. Under the law communities had to find time for new activities like political meetings of womens' and youth associations, neighbourhood groups, literacy campaigns, militia training etc.... One EPI assessment report (in three different Regions) showed a default rate ranging from 12.1% to 48%. For mothers whilst fulfilling their civil duties, did not have the time to bring their children for vaccination. A supervisory team from the Ministry of Health to the Regions of Arsi and Bale noted that the older children took the younger children to vaccination centres because of parents' commitment elsewhere. It is estimated that political participation takes about 2% of the community's time budget (Table 1).

Up to now, we discussed how people divide their time. But the community when it seeks to utilize health services encounters many obstacles which increase the waste of time. Some of these are:

8. DIALECTS AND COMMUNICATIONS

Ethiopia is a country with a population of about 30 million composed of over 10 ethnic groups, speaking over 200 languages and dialects. Language barriers and poor understanding of cultural values frustrate both health personnel and the community. The request for transfers and the grievances connected with them occupy a considerable amount of time of Ministry of Health officials.

Ethiopia is a country with 1.2 million square kilometres traversed by mountains, valleys and deserts. It has only 10, 519 kilometres of all-weather roads, 550 kilometres of railroad, a small airline and limited radio telecommunications. The communication problem is immense. Over 85% of the population lives 30 kilometres or more from an all-weather road. Travelling must be on horseback, mule or on foot, when it is possible at all. The Southern regions are not accessible during the heavy rains and the temperature in the Danakil area is unbearable during the hot season.

The absence of radios or newspapers in most rural communities creates additional barriers against a flow of new ideas and technology.

9. LIMITED COVERAGE BY HEALTH SERVICES

The health care system in Ethiopia is patterned on those found in industrialized countries. The focus is on institutional care of the sick, often in highly sophisticated hospitals, which because of their extreme expense cannot be found outside the major urban centres (21). Consequently there is little impact even on those who have access to services. After the 1974 Revolution, policies have shifted sharply from the expansion of facilities for hospital-based care towards the development of primary health care and its back-up services, but the health establishment has not yet reacted fully to the health needs of the people.

The bulk of the limited government outlays continue to go towards maintaining expensive, well-equipped hospitals manned by highly expensive medical personnel. The new government commitment will take years before it is fully reflected in the health budget. Until then the present health care coverage of less than 30% of the population will continue to be inequitable, inefficient and wasteful. One example of inequity is that a large number of people, although within the catchment area of health units, have no access to them because of their inability to pay the nominal service fee.

10. LIMITED FINANCIAL RESOURCES

Inadequacy of the budget jeopardizes the smooth running of health projects which results in a loss of faith by the people in the health programme. Those health institutions that are most affected by shortages are the local clinics and the health centres, which though built to bring services close to the rural population and thereby encourage the use of preventive and promotive services, do not enjoy the people's confidence because they are under-staffed or poorly supplied(22). Low salary, excessive work loads, poor working conditions create low morale among health personnel and further discourage community utilization. The addition of 661 general practitioners, 411 specialists, 223 pharmacists, 1856 nurses, 346 laboratory technicians, 3159 health assistants and 107 x-ray technicians will be required to staff existing health institutions.

11. BUREAUCRATIC INTENSITIVITY

In centrally designed health programmes and in cases where planning is based on inappropriate theoretical backgrounds health services not only fail to reflect the local understanding of health problems, but they fail to build a programme within the community's social and economic structure. With only one way communication of command, where the bureaucracy at the top passes the orders and those at the other end listen, the experience of those who work in the rural communities is not used. Posted in far away places without professional support, dissatisfied with their work, it is not surprising that the lot of the health worker is unhappy and unattractive to competent young people.

12. HIDDEN COSTS

Theoretically the coverage of health services is around 30% of the population (23). Because of poor communications, the time loss in travelling may exceed the possible time budget available for utilization of health services. Because of the obstacles in the delivery of health services community interest in reallocating more time for health service utilization will be minimal. Surveys and reports show that most patients visiting health facilities come from the immediate vicinity. In a study conducted in Gondar town where an antenatal service at a training health centre was free, 73% of the patients were residents of the town; 9% came from a radius of 10 km, 18% were from as far as 120 km (24), though these were cases of extreme need.

A study that is being conducted by the Statistics Division of the Ministry of Health disclosed that most of the patients of the hospitals in Addis Ababa are from the city itself, with the exception of a few with great health distress coming from further away (Table 5).

13. CONCLUSION

Health service coverage does not at present exceed 30% of the total population. One of the major reasons for lack of success in providing health services including MCH for all is that the strategy and technology of health care adopted in the past have been largely based on models developed by industrial countries without adaptation to the socio-cultural life style of the local population and the resource base of the country. As a result, health services in Ethiopia today are unequally distributed, hospital based and curative care is reaching only 5% of the total population of the country.

The main challenge of MCH programmes in the immediate future is to develop an effective health care system that is sufficiently extensive to reach all the population and is adapted to the life style of the population including their time budgets. Health programmes will then not steal community time nor be rejected as an intrusion into the socio-cultural life of the community.

The health service system should aim to minimize the time cost of utilizing services by reducing travel distance to health services or by the introduction of home visits for selective health programmes. Such innovations would be readily accepted by the community. MCH is the major element of PHC located in the community with selective and effective programmes and has great potential to achieve health and development for all by the Year 2000.

Table 1. Estimate of time budget allocations of the rural population of Tigrai Region (1980/81)

	Time budget allocation	
	Days	Percent
- Farming, herding and other productive activities	112	31
- Saturdays and Sundays (including those that coincide with monthly and annual holidays)	130[1]	28
- Market days (at least once per week)$	52	14
- Monthly church holidays (exclude those that coincide with Saturdays and Sundays)	50	14
- Annual church holidays (excluding those that coincide with Saturdays, Sundays and monthly holidays	15[2]	4
- Mortality and morbidity (excluding those that coincide with any holiday)	19[3]	5
- Political activities (excluding those that coincide with any holiday)	6[3]	2
- Birth (excluding those that coincide with holidays)	5[3]	1
- National holidays (excluding those that coincide with any other holiday or those overlooked)	3	1
Total	365	100

[1]of the 104 Saturday and Sundays, 31 days coincide with other church holidays.

[2]Annual church holidays observed number 27 but since 7 of them coincide with other holidays observed they are not included here.

[3]Estimate

[4]Rounding errors

[5]Basically covers no sleeping time activities

Table 2. Land under cultivation by the peasant population (estimate)

	1977/78	1978/79	1980/81
Land under cultivation* (millions of hectares)	5.9	6.1	6.2
Rural population** (millions)	25.7	26.3	27.0
Cultivated land per capita	0.2295	0.2319	0.2296

*Estimate by the Central Planning Supreme Council

**Based on the statistics from the Central Statistical Office

Table 3. Reasons for desiring a greater number of children

Reasons	Response %
To assist parents in work and old age	46
Appreciation of God's gift	25
Appreciation of children	22
To increase number of relatives and population	9

*Note: often the respondents gave more than one reason, hence the number of the responses exceed the number of respondents.

Source: A critical evaluation of the Family Planning Prescriptions for rural Wollo and Tigrai by Fasil G. Kiros in Ethiopian Journal of Dev. Research, Addis Ababa University, April 1970

Table 4. National holidays in Ethiopia for the year 1973 Ethiopian calendar (1980/81 EC)

Months and days	Type of holiday
September 11	Ethiopian New Year, Eritrean Reunion
September 11**	Popular Revolution Commemoration Day
September 27	The Finding of the True Cross (Meskal)
October 19	Id Al Adaha (Arafa)
January 7	Ethiopian Christmas
January 18*	Birthday of the Prophet Mohammed (Maulid)
January 19	Ethiopian Epiphany
March 2	Victory of Adwa Commemoration Day
April 6	Ethiopian Patriots Victory Day
April 24*	Ethiopian Good Friday
April 26	Ethiopian Easter
May 1	International Labour Day
August 2*	Id Alfeter (Ramadan)

Of the 13 National Holidays in 1980 one holiday falls on Saturday** while four holidays fall on Sunday*.

Table 5. Coverage of hospital services in Addis Ababa

Name of hospital	Number of patients according to where they live (%)		
	Addis Ababa	Shoa region***	other regions
Festuela*	3.2	33.2	63.6
Alert** (Leproserium)	33.2	31.1	36.1
St. Peter* (TB sanitorium)	36.1	39.9	25.0
Ghandi** (maternity)	78.6	14.0	8.4
Ethio-Swedish Pediatric Clinic**	88.3	7.1	4.6
Ethio-Swedish Pediatric Clinic*	66.2	16.0	17.8
Amanuel* (Mental)	44.8	17.5	37.7
St Paul* (General hospital)	68.9	19.1	12.0
Zewedeitu* " "	87.7	5.2	7.1
Meneliek* " "	59.9	23.1	17.0

*Inpatient **Outpatient ***Addis Ababa is the capital of Shoa

Source: From the files of the Statistics Division of the Ministry of Health, November 1980.

FOOTNOTES

(1) World Development Report, 1979. (World Bank, August 1979) p.IX.

(2) Research and Experimental Development Policy in Health, Ethiopia, (1980-84), January 1980, Draft 2; pp 3-5.

(3) National Maternal and Child Health Services in Ethiopia, Ministry of Health, August 1979.

(4) Research and Experimental Development Policy,Ibid,p.3.

(5) The Ethiopian Science and Technology Commission Health Research Council, Research and Experimental Development Policy in Health, 1980-84, January 1980, p.4.

(6) Ethiopian Peasants and Famine by Mesfin W/Mariam in the Proceedings of the Social Science Seminar, held in Nazareth, October 27-29/1978 by the Institute of University Development Research, Addis Ababa University.

(7) Tyranny of Underdevelopment by Demssie Habte, MD, December 1977.

(8) See for example Health, Sector Policy Paper of the World Bank, 1980 (World Bank, February 1980).

(9) From Report on Ethiopia Health and Family Planning Needs Assessment by R. Wiciniski, UNFPA consultant, March 1976.

(10) What we have seen during two months in a children's ward by Dr. C. Boelen in proceedings of the Fifth Health Practice Conference, Gondar June 29-July 1, 1970,pp.30-34.

(11) Prevention of maternal mortality by Dr. I.S. Bal in Proceedings of the Firth Public Health Conference Ibid, pp. 112-118.

(12) New Trends and Approaches in the Delivery of Maternal and Child Care in Health Services, Sixth Report of the WHO Expert Committee on Maternal and Child Health, Geneva 1976.

(13) For a study of vital rates see World Bank, Health Sector Policy Paper (World Bank, 1980).

(14) For discussion on the characteristics of general mortality rates through time see Macro-evaluation of Health Expenditure by Solomon Ayalew in Ethiopia Observer Vol. XVI, No.3, p.205.

(15) Paths of Development by Gunnar Myrdal (1966) in Peasant and Peasant Societies, Harmondsworth,(1971) p.414.

(16) Report of the Sub-committee on MCH & Nutrition Fourth Five Year Plan Health Sector Review, Addis Ababa, February 1973.

(17) E.C. Banfield (1958). The Moral Basis of Backward Society. The Free Press quoted in Reflections on the Concept of "Peasant Culture and Peasant Cognitive Systems" by Sutti Ortiz in Peasants and Peasant Societies ed Teodor Shanin (Middlesex: Harmondsworth, 1971).

(18) R.A. Holmberg (1967) "Algunas Relaciones la privacion psicobiologica el cambio cultural en los Andes, Amer. Indig., Vol.27 (quoted in Reflections on the concept of Peasant culture and peasant cognitive systems, op.cit).

(19) A critical evaluation of the Family Planning Prescriptions for Rural Wollo and Tigrai by Fasil G. Kirus in the Ethiopian Journal of Development Research, Addis Ababa University, April 1979, Vol. 3, No.1.

(20) See for example Political Economy of Primary Health Care Planning in Underdeveloping countries by Solomon Ayalew in a lecture presented at a seminar in the Nordic School of Public Health on Methods and Experiences in Planning for Health, Gothenburg, June 2-13, 1980.

(21) Reports from almost all health institutions show that they run out of drug budgets for at least three months of the year and that buildings are falling from lack of repair and that equipment is out of use.

(22) Health Manpower Problems in Ethiopia by Elias G. Egziabher in Ethiopian Journal of Development Research, Oct. 1979, Vol. 3, No. 2, Table 3.

(23) Ministry of Health's estimate of health service coverage is made on the assumption that a health station can provide services to 10 000 people, a health centre to 50 000 people and a rural hospital to 400 000 people. However there is no basis for this assumption.

(24) A review of 1400 ante-natal patients in Gondar by Phillis Long in Proceedings of the Fifth Public Health Practice Conference ed. Benjamin H. Bonnlander (Gondar, Ethiopia, June 29 - July 1, 1970) p. 106.

CHAPTER NINE

IDEAS FROM NEPAL FOR THE HANDICAPPED CHILD*

1. INTRODUCTION - WORDS WITHOUT ACTION

Despite the rhetoric, the IYC like many other international years has come and gone. Some countries have not even bothered to continue the momentum formally and very few have put their hands in their pockets to make a real effort. Of course the task of helping children cannot be a one-off thing, a single year or a single action. The task needs to be a continuing part of the fabric, a collective mentality in society so that the momentum continues and eventually triumphs. The problem needs to be realistically assessed and approached honestly and pragmatically. There needs to be a sound knowledge base of what people actually do and think, what they need and what they want. There needs to be mechanisms by which this knowledge can be transformed into action, especially for deprived children such as the handicapped.

* This paper has been adapted from CWCC (Child Welfare Coordination Committee) & UNICEF (Nepal), 1980, Status of Children in Nepal, Kathmandu. See especially p. 255 ff.

If all this is achieved then the best can be made out of the resources (whether internal or external) that are put into helping children, and it doesn't much matter whether we are talking about wealthy industrialised or poor rural countries.

2. NEPAL - AN ACTION CASE

Nepal is classified by the United Nations as poor country, one of those on the least developed list. But Nepal is making very great efforts for her children, efforts which began before the IYC and which are continuing after it. This paper draws on the fascinating results of efforts of the Committee of the Social Services National Coordination Council concerned with the welfare of children, established in 1979 under the chairmanship of H.R.H. Princess Sharada Shah. One of the tasks this committee has accomplished has been to study intersectorally the real needs of children, especially deprived children, such as handicapped and orphans and to make practical suggestions for improvements. The results are so interesting that they may provide ideas not only for Nepali future planning but for many other countries as well.

3. RECOMMENDATIONS FROM NEPAL - IDEALS

Our friends from Nepal write about their own situation.

"In suggesting changes and recommendations we have to consider both the expected standards and the constraints. The ideal standards should be those enduring fulfilment of the goal concerning the <u>rights of the child</u> as laid down in the U.N. Declaration of the Rights of the Child: every child has the right to:

i) affection, love and understanding;

ii) adequate nutrition and medical care;

iii) free education;

iv) a name and nationality;

v) special care, if handicapped;

vi) be among the first to receive relief in the time of disaster;

vii) learn to be a useful member of society and to develop individual abilities;

viii) be brought up in a spirit of peace and universal brotherhood;

ix) enjoy these rights, regardless of race, shelter and education for basic minimum needs.

Constraints: In Nepal, 40.5 per cent of the total population is below the age of 14 and over 40 per cent of the population falls below the poverty line. The per capita income is Rs. 1,272 per year. In practical terms, these statistics mean that the basic needs of the majority of the population have hardly been met; so special attention must be paid to the children because they are the most vulnerable group, and an integrated approach to social services/welfare in general also must be considered in view of the following constraints.

The basic constraints as identified by this study are: (i) the general public's indifferent or negative attitude towards social services in general and welfare of the handicapped in particular, (ii) lack of people's participation in social service, particularly service for the handicapped, (iii) lack of funds to establish and run institutions for child welfare in particular, and social service in general, (however it is necessary to analyse each institution's budget to pinpoint which areas require financing), (iv) lack of trained professional as well as managerial manpower to staff the institutes.

There are few institutions besides schools dealing specifically with children's welfare. Most of such institutions are in Kathmandu and only a few are located in other parts of the country. Most of these, except Samaj Kalyan Kendra, receive budget support from various foreign sources. It is clear that there has not been enough initiative to obtain community contributions. This is partly due to local financial constraints, but there are other equally pertinent reasons.

4. RECOMMENDATIONS FROM NEPAL - LONG TERM MEASURES

a) Efforts must be made at all levels within and outside the Government to change the people's attitude towards social service in general, and towards helping the handicapped in particular.

To ensure country participation, people's attitudes must be changed. The general attitude towards the handicapped children and orphans that their present (unfortunate) condition is the result of their past life, i.e. of "Karma" and again because of Karma, they are those unfortunate people who have to earn their living by helping and taking care of such children. This is apparently the reason why people do not help or are not associated with those less fortunate ones in society.

There are also superstitions about the handicapped; there is a belief for instance that blind children should not live with non-blind children, because they may go blind simply through association with them. We were told that these beliefs are strongly held, especially by religious-minded people. Except for Paropakar, none of the institutions we visited had any local community members sufficiently involved nor were any efforts made in them to involve the local people. The public must be made to realise that these people are handicapped due to no faults of their own, and that it is normal for any society to have a certain percentage of children handicapped or orphaned. The public must also be made to realise that every human being, normal or otherwise has a right to food, shelter, education and a decent standard of living and a right to be treated properly. The public must be motivated to show empathy towards the unfortunate and to consider it their obligation to help their less fortunate fellow citizens. Nepalese citizens at the highest level in the existing political, economic and social organizations can educate and inspire the public via radio, magazines, newspapers, documentaries, public speeches, the local panchayats and by concrete examples. Non-governmental organizations, such as the Chambers of Commerce, Boy Scouts, National Development Service of Tribhuvan University, Red Cross and the likes can and should be active in this respect. Such organizations could educate the public, help raise funds and involve themselves in the affairs of the social service institutions.

b) Efforts must be made to involve the local community in social services and in raising local contributions, both financial and otherwise, to institutions dealing with less fortunate children as well as to the handicapped in general.

The local community's active involvement in such institutions is vital for their successful functioning, expansion and improvement. Community participation is required to obtain funds for the institution as the Government at present cannot finance all the institutions, nor can the international agencies do so. Even if institutions could be financed with foreign aid, the community's involvement is necessary in order to integrate normal and handicapped children through educational and extra-curricular activities.

c) Special efforts must be directed towards educating the parents and family members of the handicapped children so that they no longer feel ashamed of these children. Helping the handicapped children to contribute to the family's income by giving them vocational training and providing them with jobs is a step towards changing the family's attitudes. We were told that the parents' attitudes towards and their treatment of children improved after the children received vocational training and were able to contribute to the family's income.

We found that most of the family members did not do much to help the handicapped children, who were generally left alone and even maltreated. For most families, the residential facilities offered by institutions were a big relief both financially and otherwise. Parents and family members must be taught methods of communicating with, and caring for, such as braille, speaking to the dumb, understanding the deaf, handling mentally retarded children, etc. One incentive could be to arrange for compulsory paid leave for the employed family members attending such training or to pay nominal stipends for those attending.

d) Efforts must also be made to change the people's attitude towards orphans, and towards the adoption of orphans. Because of the strong emphasis laid on the family or caste background of the children, the Nepalese have not yet started to adopt legally orphans in such numbers as we could. The few Nepalese who adopt children insist on strict confidentiality in order to hide the child's family background, and this is not always to the long-term benefit of the child. Furthermore, there are other factors restricting the adoption of Nepalese children by Nepalese, but they can be minimised by means of legal action.

e) It is necessary to ensure integration of the handicapped and the normal children. The orphans attend local schools so there is some amount of integration at this level as they have daily contact with the children who have parents. As for the handicapped, only the Laboratory School has integrated the blind both in the classrooms and in the residence. In depth research is required to find out if integration is and has been beneficial to the normal as well as the handicapped children. While the blind children claimed to be quite happy with the integration, the non-blind children were said to be not very happy with it. The teachers concerned with the blind students claimed that the blind suffered academically and that there should be separate institutions for the blind. They agreed that integration would benefit both the blind and the non-blind socially. Even if it were not possible to have common residential facilities or classrooms it would still be possible to have integration of the children at the public level. The handicapped children and the orphans must be "brought out in public" and not hidden away. Arranging common activities with the normal children from other institutions (say once a week) could be the first step towards the children's acceptance of the handicapped and the orphans into their groups.

Schools could organize quiz contests, games and cultural activities in which these children could participate. People from organizations like the Boy Scouts and Girl Guides, Junior Red Cross, etc. could visit these institutions and organise games/cultural activities or just stay there and talk to the handicapped and the orphans. This will be an educational experience for both as the normal children will learn to accept and understand the unfortunate children and the handicapped and the orphans will feel accepted and learn to interact with the normal children.

f) More people must be trained to take care of the handicapped and the orphans. The existing institutions lack adequately trained personnel and so are unable to give appropriate and professional care to these children. More trained and professional people will be required not only for the existing institutions but also for any new institution which will be opened.

For this, an institute should be opened in Nepal to train people in social welfare as well as teachers for the blind, the deaf and other handicapped children. Trainers for such an institute should be appropriately educated in Nepal or outside.

g) Rehabilitation of the orphans and handicapped children should be properly planned and implemented. At present, most of the institutions do not have any fixed plans for rehabilitation, although some do find jobs for their children.

Rehabilitation is essential for the orphans who have nobody to turn to for help. Institutions themselves must do more to find appropriate jobs for them and also keep regular contact with them to ensure their progress and well-being.

In order to ensure that these people lead as normal a life as possible, appropriate arrangements could also be made for their marriage.

h) Provision of jobs for the orphans and the handicapped is also an essential long-term measure which requires immediate attention. While recognizing the fact that over 40 per cent of the population in Nepal falls below the poverty line and that they need jobs, the orphans and the handicapped need jobs equally urgently, especially since most of these children belong also to the lower class. We recommend that the possibility of tax incentives to industries employing orphans and the handicapped at regular salary scales in regular jobs be studied. The government's resettlement projects could also give due consideration to settling orphans on resettlement lands.

Giving vocational training to those children in knitting, tailoring, carpet weaving, carpentry, typing and other trades will enable them to work. Clerical work in the banks and offices could also be handled by some. The idea would be to accommodate these orphans and the handicapped, to the maximum possible extent.

5. RECOMMENDATIONS FROM NEPAL - SHORT-TERM MEASURES

We found that many of the institutions could not function effectively due to their organizational structure and communication difficulties. We recommend some changes:

a) Specialists and people trained in caring for the handicapped must be on the boards to represent the special interests of the children. Some of the heads of institutions should be on the boards to decide policies. The present board members are often too busy in other things or they lack the knowledge to understand the peculiar problems of these children and yet they are involved in making policies.

b) The heads of the institutions must have to be delegated authority and responsibility and the corresponding accountability so they can manage the institutions more effectively. A precise job description must be given to the staff members so they know what their duties and responsibilities are.

c) The staff members must be given short, compact courses in child welfare as a stop-gap measure while some are properly trained. This could be achieved by some form of intensive in-service training.

d) The facilities for the children are not adequate. We suggest that more attention be paid to their emotional, recreational and medical needs. To ensure special attention to their emotional needs, child guidance counsellors and child psychologists have to be employed to guide the children. It is a well-documented fact that early deprivation (either physical or emotional) have a long-lasting ill-effect in the child's life style. We hold the view that adequate food, shelter and fancy "educational toys" alone will not suffice for their growth and development.

6. RECOMMENDATIONS FROM NEPAL - FINANCES

As a short-term measure, the finance for running the institutions should be generated as much as possible from the public through such means as lotteries, charity shows, donations, improved tax administration. All-round improvement of the present tax administration would go a long way even under existing tax laws, in alleviating financial constraints. Guthi funds should also be more extensively allocated for special child welfare. Such means could supply most of the finances for the daily expenditure of institutions. In order to ensure public confidence in charitable efforts, accounts should be made public as part of the fund-raising efforts and auditing provided by independent auditors appointed by the Social Services National Coordination Council. Further, various international agencies could be approached to obtain funds to construct buildings, equipment, etc. but institutional and self-reliance and proper management must always be stressed.

7. RECOMMENDATIONS FROM NEPAL - PLANNING, SUPERVISION AND COORDINATION

The setting up of the Social Services National Coordination Council under the chairmanship of Her Majesty Queen Aishwarya in 1977 filled a large void in the institutional make up in matters pertaining to social welfare in general and the well-being of the orphans, the mentally and physically handicapped and the socially disadvantaged groups on account of their age, sex or caste. The royal leadership being provided by the Queen is serving as a major catalytic event in bringing about awareness among the people on the rights of the disadvantaged groups of society and the duties of the stage, and of the privileged and able-bodied citizens towards them. Much more, however, remains to be done in the areas of planning, supervision and coordination if existing institutions are to be made more effective in securing their individual goals; and also if the summation of their collective efforts is to have a greater dynamic impact on the general well-being of the Kingdom's children.

A major weakness in national planning has been its failure to specify target groups and as a consequence, programmes pertaining to children are neither integrated nor comprehensive enough to cater to many of their basic needs. Needs of special significance for child development are also those in such areas as sports, recreation, sanitation and public hygiene, which remain particularly neglected by the national planning process. Where, however, basic needs are being provided for, as in areas like education, health, drinking water, food production etc. it would appear that the thrust of these past development efforts has been insufficient on account of poor resource mobilization and a low level of absorptive capacity in the bureaucratic structure. Planning must, therefore, address itself more fully towards locating and developing alternative institutions for formulation, implementation and evaluation of plans and engender better budgetary allocation (annually) for children's welfare programmes. Further, improved coordination at the plan formulation stage will go a long way to enhancing coordination generally if the present technique of economic sector planning could be integrated by the National Planning Commission to incorporate social planning techniques to assess the extent of basic needs being rendered for the various target groups of the population, especially in our case, the children.

Although the number of non-educational institutions catering to children's welfare is limited in the range of needs served and they are heavily localized in the capital city, adequate supervision by concerned authorities is vitally necessary for institutional development and growth. Beside supervision over their financial transactions through the introduction of auditing practices, it is necessary to inculcate supervisory habits based on well-stipulated standards and norms. This is a responsibility which the Social Services National Coordination Council could fruitfully be engaged in as part of its research publicity and information endeavours. As pointed out in the study, many of the existing institutions suffer from the lack of trained and qualified manpower. Any effort to develop standards and norms should, therefore, take due cognizance of specifying not only standards and norms for physical environment and facilities but also manpower qualifications and their salary and other service conditions. Similarly another method of enhancing coordination would be to facilitate communications between existing institutions towards this, the Council could support the publication of newsletters, journals etc. which could incorporate the goings-on in the diverse institutions. Also, it could fund short-term inservice and institutional training programmes for the social workers. A paramount task which deserves high priority in the work of the Council pertains to how local community participation could be accelerated to help meet children's needs in general. Much will depend on the leadership provided by the panchayat and social workers at the grass-roots level. Bureaucratic efforts too need strengthening. Towards this end, it would be desirable to have a person at the district level to give full time attention to child development and welfare in the envisaged District Administration Plan of His Majesty's Government.

The special Education Division of the Ministry of Education should not only be concerned with the provision of finance but also enlarge its function to involve supervision and inspection of existing institutions concerned with development and welfare of Nepalese children. An Annual Inspection Report on the status of such schools should invariably be presented to the concerned Ministry for scrutiny before bringing it to the notice of the general public. Particular emphasis needs to be given to supervision and inspection of institutions in remote areas of the Kingdom. Further the

Division should serve as the focal point in the bureaucratic setup to undertake regular surveys to assess children's needs and to prepare projects for funding through national and foreign agencies. This division should also initiate the removal of legal provisions in the diverse legal instruments which debar the employment and representation of the dumb, deaf and disabled persons from being able to contribute to national social, political and economic development processes. Finally this Division could profitably initiate measures to have Tribhuvan University develop curricula for social work".

8. THE LESSONS OF NEPAL FOR OTHER COUNTRIES

If self-awareness is the first step in achieving goals, then Nepal has made an important beginning. The main lessons are that there is a need for people themselves to change their attitudes in the long term, especially towards very deprived children, such as the handicapped and the orphaned. There is a need for public support morally and financially. There is a need for more communication and cooperation. In this, the role of the outsider, of foreigners and foreign aid, may not be very useful, even counterproductive. The health and welfare of children depend on dynamics within societies, even within individuals. Nepal has, unlike many societies, a blueprint and it remains to be seen how many people will take heed of it, even now as we have another International Year, focussing activities on the handicapped.

CHAPTER TEN

RETHINKING CHILDREN - A NEW DIMENSION FOR INTERNATIONAL DEVELOPMENT ACTION

1. PROBLEMS

The International Year of the Child highlighted the sad plight of many children. Throughout the world, but particularly in the developing countries, there are as many as 500 million children living in conditions of absolute poverty.

In 1975 (1) something like 70% of these children lived in rural areas (in Africa the figure was nearer 80%). Many of the children in urban areas who lived in slums and squatter settlements had come recently from rural areas, and the numbers were increasing rapidly. Of the approximately 125 million children born each year in the world, at least 12 million die before their first birthday(44), and of these deaths 10 million (2) are in the developing world. In Asia, the expectation of life is around 57 at birth; in Africa, it is only 46(3). There is widespread malnutrition.

There are estimates of 500 million children who encounter sickness or disabling disease brought on by, or aggravated by protein calorie malnutrition(4). Malnutrition is, too, the major causal factor in low birthweights and high infant mortality. Bad housing(5), bad water unhealthy environments, inadequate access to medical services all add to the toll of morbidity and mortality. There are large numbers of handicapped children, perhaps 173 million, partly realted to malnutrition. The ubiquity of war and disaster has left in its shadow many needy children.

If, in situations of poverty the health of children is bad, most children are also deprived of education. It is estimated(6) that only one third of school-age children in the developing world are in fact receiving education. For some categories, e.g. female teenagers, the proportion is even lower(7), and even the children in school receive an inappropriate education or drop out.

Many school-age children, perhaps as much as another third, are at work(8). Although there is sometimes valuable training for later life on the job, much child labour is exploitative, unhealthy, illegal, degrading and demeaning. In some situations, children work 80 hours a week, often in dangerous and insanitary conditions.

Then there are another third of the school-age children who seem to be unemployed as well as uneducated, abandoned and idle, often drifting into lives of crime and unhappiness.

The situation of the youth of the world is different, but still abject and poverty stricken. In the developing world, only 0.6% enrol in tertiary institutions; many of the estimated 40% who are unemployed are young people(9).

In short, in a world of poverty, many children are the most poor, whilst many rural children, even more neglected because of an urban bias in development and planning, are the poorest of the poor. In the seventies, it became widely recognized that the eradication of poverty and the fulfilment of basic needs was the major goal of international action. However, for a variety of reasons this huge and chronic problem could not easily be resolved. The eighties may well be a period when poverty-oriented and basic needs approaches need to have a sharper focus, more refined objectives, and concrete procedures concentrating on social groups such as women and children.

Two things are particularly disturbing about these figures on children. They reveal enormous problems, but are probably very conservative. Statistics in developing countries are often only estimates. A first major challenge, in fact, is to find timely and acceptable modes of collecting vital statistics and other measurements needed to provide the indicators and signposts for planned future development.

The second and much more disturbing fact is that the situation in many countries is not improving, and may, in fact, be deteriorating, despite an awareness of the problem since the end of the second world war and considerable efforts by development agencies, nationally and internationally.

There are many reasons for this situation. In an interdependent world, the chain of causality is long. To explain why a baby dies in a remote village, it is necessary to consider such diverse factors as the structure of the world economy, the bureaucratic difficulties of agencies, nationally and internationally, as well as more immediate problems of water, housing nutrition, medical services, etc. in the village itself.

If the problems are dimly perceived, then the solutions, and, particularly, the effects of them, are even less well understood(10). Global strategies have not dealt adequately with global complexeties, whilst solutions coming in at critical points have led to all kinds of unexpected consequences.

Much development aid is dissipated because there is not a clear and long-term focus around which there can be consensual planning. Too often plans are vitiated because they are set in short term economic contexts and because they are destroyed by political struggles.

2. SOLUTIONS - THE DEPRIVED CHILD AS A DEVELOPMENT FOCUS

In many senses, the deprived child can be seen as an ideal focus for development. The children of today will be the adults of the year 2000, and are, therefore, an essential part of a long-term strategy that prepares the way for development for all and seeks to prevent the mortality, morbidity and deprivation which is so prevalent amongst today's children. Around the child unite all development sectors and disciplines. The child, as the International Year of the Child demonstrated so clearly, is politically neutral and a unanimously approved target group. Finally, children are an entry point which allows programmes to reach and involve the adult. The problem of the child cannot be separated from the development problems of women and the family, and so there is extra support for this important new international direction.

A strong case can be made for the child as the focus of rural and slum development. Certainly there are existing mechanisms, some work has been done, and there is a conciousness of the problem. But, in reality, the child has had a low profile as a specific target in the real politik of national and international strategies and politics. Certainly, there has been a major international year, the International Year of the Child, which has generated much publicity and goodwill, and there are other years which include deprived children (e.g. the Year of the Disabled, 1981, Youth 1985). Despite possible long-term beneficial effects of present programmes, there is a desperate need for a rethinking on ways of increasing present effectivness so that the problems we have talked about are mitigated. A recent World Bank publication talks about the invisible(11) woman in development, and much the same comments could be made about the child. There were many expressions of support: for example, at the UN General Assembly which concluded the IYC activities. There may be political consensus, but there is not political will relative to other priorities. There is a UN agency, UNICEF, but its history has been one of funding ad hoc projects and with some exceptions it has not broken through into the key international sectors. In some countries, children seem to have become located in the realm of innocuous female power structures, and often the First Lady is the key person in promoting activities for the child.

There are few countries which have politically powerful government departments or statutory bodies concerned specifically with children. Activities concerned with children are often spread across a bureaucracy in which there is too seldom cooperation and coordination. Fragmentation has led to much complexity, which, in turn, has created inefficiency. Even the exchange of information is difficult, and although much is known about the child in many scattered pockets, much of this is not generally known because the information is not made visible, shared and utilized(12).

Part of the reason for the low profile of the child in politics and planning is the weak emphasis on the child in the theoretical models of the dominant development disciplines, notably economics, which tend to have more abstract kinds of orientations(43). There were several tendencies which created this emphasis. First, because of the importance attached in the sixties and seventies to relating population to development, there was a bias towards theories which stressed population and fertility control. Recently, the pendulum has begun to swing to an emphasis on mortality(13) and its prevention. Infant mortality and the expectancy of life, together with literacy, have become the key indicators of the quality of life(14). There is evidence to suggest that this humanistic interpretation is much nearer that of grass roots opinion where the child is a central object in folk development theories, and the prevalence of infant mortality a major reason for population behaviour(15). But probably the gravest fault of the theories is the relative absence of thoroughgoing interdisciplinary work, and even more significantly, there are too few mechanisms by which theories can be translated into action.

3. REVIEW OF ACTION - THE BASIC MOVEMENT

It is true that some international action has been taken even if the child has never been in centre stage. The history of recent endeavours in the specialized agencies and thinking in many developed countries has emphasized combatting poverty by concentrating on basic needs, Primary Health Care and basic services, building up wherever possible using a country's own resources. The object has been a high degree of self reliance and popular participation, of internally-generated development rather than externally imposed programmes.

Although these have been pious hopes rather than concrete achievements, some progress has been made. Certainly all the UN agencies have moved in recent years part way along this road - in what might be called the Basic movement, i.e. where basic needs, services, primary health care, access to land, food, etc. have been key elements. For FAO, the World Conference on Agrarian Reform and Rural Development has provided the framework for new approaches to rural development in which the country's own Centres for Integrated Rural Development will play an important part(16). In the WCAARD Programme of Action, of great importance is better access to land, other resources and markets, the integration of women as well as more appropriate international actions. But the child has received much less attention in the WCARRD deliberations. Interagency efforts such as the FAO, WHO, UNICEF, World Bank proposal to mount an action programme for the rural mother and child through the CIRDs has been slow moving.

The vicissitudes of this project are a vignette of the sorts of problems which any international project faces. It was set up after informal discussions in late 1979 between deeply-interested staff members at the FAO, WHO, UNICEF and the World Bank. But there were difficulties in getting recognition, in-house, partly because agencies fears of offending each other or of impinging on each other's territory. The project became caught up, to some degree, in the administrative snarl of the ACC(45). There were, therefore, difficulties in bringing in the countries, but it was something of Catch 22 situation because country support would have given the agencies a mandate as well as a stimulus. The project tended, therefore, to fall between all the stools, even though there were donors who were anxious to support it. The long and involuted chains of communication meant long delays too in the countries, especially in the establishement of the nationally-sponsored integrated rural development centres and networks. There were difficulties in making them genuinely intersectoral enterprises or bringing them into effective contact with other networks such as the health development networks. Nonetheless, the project is moving ahead. Four countries in Asia have shown interest, an integrated rural development network is planned for Africa and nearly 30 countries are involved, whilst there are similar moves in Latin America and the Middle East.

For WHO/UNICEF, an interest in promoting the welfare of the rural child can be seen as part of the doctrine of Primary Health Care most clearly enunciated at the 1978 UNICEF/WHO Meeting in Alma-Ata, which, itself, drew on earlier work on basic needs and services(17). There were 8 pillars in the Alma-Ata declaration which were the minimum inclusions in a PHC package(18), viz.: health education, proper nutrition, safe water and basic sanitation, maternal and child health (MCH) care, including family planning, immunization against major infectious diseases, prevention and control of locally-endemic diseases, appropriate treatment of common diseases and injuries, the provision of essential drugs. All the Alma-Ata principles have the most important repercussions for child health and welfare in rural settings, and it has been claimed that one reason why the child is not mentioned more at WHO is because everything revolves around the child. But PHC has proved an elusive and costly hope. It is estimated that to achieve PHC, for example, would require a tripling of external aid(19) as well as a maximum internal commitment most countries cannot or will not afford.

In addition, UNICEF has taken over the roles of the IYC Secretariat, in conjunction with a new consultative group drawn from a wide range of agencies.

All this has strengthened UNICEF's long standing interests in providing basic services for children(20). The following 5 characteristics have been emphasized in the idea of basic services:

i) active community participation;

ii) the use of suitably-trained, local persons, part-time or full-time chosen by the community to work there;

iii) the use of a substantially higher number of auxillary staff, in combination with those in (ii) above so releasing professional people to be trainers, supervisors, programme directors, etc.;

iv) application of technology appropriate to the local, social, cultural and economic conditions;

v) contributions from the community to help finance basic services in cash, kind, labour and other services.

It is recognized that the most important factor is the will of the community concerned(21).

Certainly, the UNICEF initiative had born fruit in a number of specific case studies in countries. For example, through the United Nations Social Welfare and Development Centre for Asia and the Pacific - case studies on methods and techniques of developing basic rural community services for children had been carried out in four countries - Indonesia, Korea, Malysia and the Philippines(22). Through the International Council for Educational Development Essex, there were studies on CBIRD(22a) which was not so much a model, but a flexible strategy as Coombs described it for achieving community-based integrated rural development. CBIRD and related case studies were carried out in Bangladesh, Sri Lanka, India, Indonesia, Thailand and South Korea.

Since 1973, after Mr. McNamara's famous poverty speech, the Bank has vigorously pursued(23) a poverty approach to rural development. The emphasis on the child may be seen as a refinement of this by concentrating on a specific target group, although there have been few concrete programmes.

The ILO and UNESCO have similar programmes concentrating on basic services, basic needs and grass roots initiatives with regard to the child. The UNESCO/UNICEF programmes to study basic services and learning priorities is a good example(24). UNESCO has recently taken the initiative in convening important meetings on the needs of the child and the contribution the social sciences can make. The former meetings has stressed a desperate need for international cooperation(25).

The ILO has widespread interests in the problem of child labour, as well as more general interests in rural poverty(26). The basic needs approach (perhaps the most influential of all the basic philosophies) was first presented at the ILO World Employment Conference in 1976, though it drew on the work of at least a decade in many institutions(27). Although there were varying interpretations of the doctrine, there were a number of common characteristics. Covered were not only material needs (food, shelter, clothing, sanitation), public and communal services (education, health), but, also human rights, participation, self reliance(28), etc. with some attempt to establish minimal standards. The approach was intended to be flexible in space and time, varying from country to country with the hope that the goals would be accomplished within a generation. Finally, and most significantly, there was an emphasis on the need for "structural transformation" and a "redistribution of political power"(29).

A number of criticisms of basic needs and the other basic movements can be made however. Some third-world countries were concerned that despite the development from below rhetoric, this was still a top down exercise, which, moreover, tended to enshrine poverty by having only minimal aspirations. The Group of 77, now well over a 100 developing nations, saw basic needs as a diversion from the central need(30) to create a new international economic order, and, in fact, a means of maintaining dependency. There were fears that the implications of structural transformation would, at worst, create revolutionary situations and were, at least interferences in the internal affairs of countries. There were feelings that many elements were emergency ad hoc projects. Naturally, too, there was opposition from those who saw the basic movements as opposed to conventional economic growth. Emmerrij(31), amongst others, has argued that these views were fallacies, but they were still widely believed. And there were many ambivalances too (over the population question, for example), as well as great difficulties in translating the rhetoric into reality, in particular in achieving or stimulating intersectoral coordination at both the international and national levels. Despite the momentum of the IYC, the child figured little in the debates in the UN General Assembly in August 1980 on the New International Development Strategy, though there was a mention in the influential Brandt Report.

If the UN had tended to overlook the child, the NGO movement was very much more active. The idea for the IYC itself had, in fact, come from Canon Moerman of the International Catholic Child Bureau in Geneva, and the NGOs were largely responsible for carrying on any momentum of the IYC. The Dag Hammarskjöld Foundation had published a seminal book(32) on the child in the mid-1970s which was having an increasing and deep effect in Africa and beyond. The NGOs were major activists too in the important argument over infant feeding and the attempt to control, through a Code, the activities of the multinationals in advertising and selling infant food formula.

The new emphasis on the child may be seen in some ways as an extension of the basic movement, and a beginning towards a new international social order. Many of the principles in the basic movement of the focus on the poor, the emphasis on self-reliance, popular will, etc. are accepted. But the idea is taken much farther, and it is also hoped the kinds of objections that have been raised to the "basic" movement may be in part answered. For example, by choosing the deprived child as a specific target group, much of the political argument is avoided. The child is neutral ground, and, in a sense, structural transformation and redistribution takes place through the child, even if it is a long-term process. Projects would not only be emergency and ad hoc measures, but as part of a continuing long-term strategy, a major vehicle of achieving health, education, food, etc. for all by the year 2000 when today's children will be adults. Projects would put much more emphasis on local, country initiatives. The object is not really so much to work through, but from country level institutions, and in this way strengthening them. There is too very little ambivalence over the population and development issue. The child philosophy would stand squarely in the new trend which emphasizes mortality (and particularly infant mortality) control rather than fertility control(33). The basic movement has produced a great many theoretical studies: the object here would be to move more rapidly into the action field.

Of course, there remain dilemmas and difficulties. The interface with economic growth is still problematical. The problem of the restructuring of the world economy is still a basic underlying factor and should, as the Brandt Report has emphasized, be a priority. The redistribution of resources in favour of the child could be a start in this direction. There is still a confrontation between the internationals and multinationals, and perhaps what is called for is an extension of the dialogue of the kind that WHO/UNICEF initiated in 1979 in Geneva with regard to infant feeding(34).

New ground needs to be broken by looking at the question of rationalizing and operationalizing the different agency thrusts. In a definite sense, a critical failing of basic needs, services, primary health care, etc. programmes has not necessarily been the philosophy, but the difficulties of getting different agencies and sectors to work together at <u>all</u> levels.

4. THE NEW UN ROLE

Despite the long and deep involvement of the UN family in action for the rural child, there is a great need for cooperation, coordination and more positive directions. There is certainly evidence that the countries themselves are becoming increasingly dissatisfied with a situation where, in many instances, agencies are competing with each other, and, certainly, are more worried about poaching and trespassing on each other's territory than getting on with the job. The existing mechanisms for coordination (such as the ACC) are complex and cumbersome.

The United Nations role should be catalytic and animatory towards the countries, responding to their demands and requests. One of the most important roles, therefore, that the agencies could play is to provide valid and useful information, and generally to assist in the process of communication, both TCDC and North/South. It seems ironical that in a world which has developed relatively low cost, highly effective communication systems, that the exchange of knowledge should be one of the weakest links in the chain.

In addition, the United Nations family could provide a much more flexible pool of resources (including funding) and expertise which countries could draw on. Many countries, and indeed institutions and individuals are actively seeking support and the long experience of the United Nations should be invaluable. At all points, countries would be encouraged to set up and implement programmes themselves.

Although the United Nations role should be low key and retiring, there are also important global roles to play. Even though much is known about the general nature of the problems of the child, and even though in the past research has too often been an excuse for inaction, there is still a need for action research, as some of the mechanisms in the basic, critical relationships are not well understood. There is a desperate shortage of accurate statistics with which to construct new indicators to assist in the planning process. There is particularly very little knowledge about the best ways any theoretical knowledge can be translated into action. What may be needed is an intensive, but inexpensive case study research programme in a small number of countries (perhaps of the rapid appraisal(35) type), which could provide not only typical answers to some of these problems but also, models and guidelines of how best to carry out the kind of shoestring ongoing research that is vital to the planning process.

The list of priority research topics is long. But most countries are not starting from scratch, even if few countries have anything like an adequate statistical and documentary record. In many cases, critical materials are missing. For example, it is becoming widely agreed that a key indicator for planning is infant mortality(36), but this needs an adequate birth registration system. Much work needs to be done on indirect estimation statistics, sample surveys, etc. A UN role may well be to encourage an international campaign to record as many births as possible in one year in selected areas.

The United Nations family could also assist from its considerable experience by convening international fora, consultations, etc., by generally providing countries with models of training programmes(37) and, indeed, of the curricula itself. Ideas have been floated in WHO of utilizing much more open learning techniques and the media, including satellite transmissions(38), both in training "practitioners" and a much wider outreach to the public. New innovative mechanisms are needed, such as the child-to-child programme(39). Again, all these activities have been actively demanded by the countries themselves.

Another area which has been neglected is the perception by the people themselves (including the children themselves) of development problems and of specific wants and aspirations. The classification of basic needs tends to be those needs which bureaucrats in agencies remote from the villages consider to be the most significant, and it may be more useful to look now at basic wants, for people rarely seem to want what they need. Of critical importance are the ways in which scarce resources are used for development. Official priorities often put economic growth or military expenditures as first priorities. The latter especially is not usually a popular wish and as far as children are concerned, war and its associated phenomena is one of the gravest threats to well being. But even the relatively large expenditures on health and education may not benefit people as much as the planners in central government feel. Health services may not reach peripheral areas, and even if there are aims of universal education, these aims are seldom realized. As we have said, studies have shown that the average(40) child is a working child, and the needs and wants of this child should be the central focus of development action and expenditure.

The research could be of two kinds. First, there is a need to establish what are the causal patterns and consequences of the major factors in any community situation including, in particular, the effects of the introduction of new technologies or behaviour. Very often the bad effects of development have been the unintended consequences of good intentions. The ILO studies on child labour have demonstrated how complex and specific, patterns of causality can be, and demonstrate clearly that if planning and legislation are to be effective, they need to have a flexibility that can only come from a very clear picture of this kind of complexity.

Secondly, although there is a great deal of information extant, much is buried away and scattered. An essential task is, therefore, to make this research visible and hence useable. This analysis, which might also yield the bonus of hindsights, is far more preferable than new research in which there is only a hazy notion of what to look for. The process of stocktaking needs a systematic checklist of information. The UN family could well help by constructing a classification which would allow a rapid and logical ordering of the data and would encourage, also, easy international comparability. At the moment, most attention has been focused on the need for quantitative data such as statistical indicators, but, in the long term, as in other branches of comparative studies, more valuable insights and clues to interpreting the quantitative data will have to come from qualitative documentary material. This process could be speeded by methods such as rapid rural appraisal, where approximate materials are gathered in very quickly(41).

The United Nations role might well extend more into legal and advocacy questions. As the pioneering WHO/UNICEF(42) initiative in convening a meeting on infant and young child feeding clearly showed, there is a very great need to bring industry, NGOs and governments, as well as international agencies into situations of dialogue about controversial issues. Such initiatives may well produce codes of conduct or conventions that would protect more adequately the rights of the child.

There are some who doubt whether it is within the capacity of the UN system to achieve the necessary coordination and momentum. Alternatives are being suggested which would call for a relatively independent body, rather as the Brandt Report has suggested. Whatever the result of these debates, it is certain that the problems of the child need to be attacked on many fronts and the widest range of possibilities should be examined.

FOOTNOTES

(1) UN Population Division, WP/54, McHale 1979 5 below p.4 and 18 for the following figures. We follow here the UN practice of using country definitions of what is urban, which, in some countries, may be as much as 50,000 people per settlement.

(2) WHO - 1980 - Towards a Better Future - Maternal and Child Health, Geneva, p.7.

(3) Abel-Smith B - 1978 - Poverty, Development and Health Policy - WHO, Geneva, Ch. 1

(4) FAO - 1970 - Lives in Peril - Rome, p.7, 1977 - Fourth World Food Survey, Part 2, McHale et al - 1979 -gives 230 million as undernourished

(5) McHale et al - 1979 - gives 417 million (bad housing), 590 million without access to safe water, 604 million without access to effective medical care - McHale J. 1979 - Tomorrows Children - Washington.

(6) UNESCO - 1980 - Conference on the Needs of the Child - Paris

(7) Population Reference Bureau - World's Children Data Sheet - Washington - 1980

(8) See Defence for Children - 1981 - Child Labour - Geneva Soon Young Yoon has claimed that all children work in Asia - see her Developments Orphans - 1978 - UNAPDI - Bangkok

(9) See United Nations - 1979 - Report on the World Social Situation - New York

(10) For one attempt, see Hunter G - 1978 - Agricultural Development and the Rural Poor - London, ODI

(11) World Bank - 1979 - Women and Development - Washington

(12) The IYC Discussion Paper on Rural Children, p.l. talks of only fleeting images

(13) See the papers of the CECRED/WHO Meeting on Socio-Economic Factors and Mortality, Geneva, July 1980

(14) e.g. Morris D. Morris - 1979 - Measuring the Conditions of the World's Poor - Washington, Streeten P and Hicks N - 1980 - Indicators of Development - The Search for a Basic Needs Yardstick - Development Digest, Vo.18, No.1

(15) cf David Pitt - 1979 - Social Synamics of Development - Oxford - Pergamon

(16) See FAO - 1979 - World Conference on Agrarian Reform and Rural Development, Rome

(17) cf Djukanovic V and Mach EP - 1975 - Alternative Approaches to Meeting Basic Health Needs in Developing Countries - UNICEF/WHO - Geneva.

(18) Formulating Health Strategies for All by the Year 2000 - WHO - Geneva - 1979

(19) see S. C. Joseph and S. S. Russell - 1980 - in Health Population in Developing Countries - Social Science and Medicine - vol. 14c, page 121-9

(20) See Assignment Children - no. 37 - January-March 1977

(21) see UNICEF - 1979 - Joint WHO/UNICEF Meeting on Infant and Young Child Feeding, Geneva

(22) See UNSWDCAP - 1980 - Cross National Analysis of Four Case Studies Manila (Preliminary Draft)

(22a) Brandt V S R and Ji Woong Cheong - 1979 - CBIRD is defined in Planning from the Bottom Up - ICED - Essex

(23) See e.g. Srinivasan T - 1977 - Development, Poverty and Basic Needs, World Bank Reprint Series, No. 76, or Staff Paper 309, etc. Health, Including Child Health is discussed in the Health, Sector Policy Paper -February 1980

(24) e.g. IBE - 1978 - Basic Services for Children - a continuing search for learning priorities - UNESCO - Paris

(25) UNESCO - Interagency Consultation on the Needs of the Child - Paris - 13 June 1980 - Final Report

(26) e.g. ILO - 1977 - Poverty and Landlessness in Rural Asia - World Employment Programme - ILO - Geneva

(27) See ILO - 1976 - Employment Growth and Basic Needs -A One World Problem - Geneva. cf Dag Hammarskjöld Foundation - 1975 - What now - another development -Uppsala. Tinbergen J et al - 1976 - Reshaping the International Order - Amsterdam/New York - Dutton. Bariloche Foundation - 1976 - Catastrophe or New Society - A Latin American World Model - Buenos Aires

(28) See the January 1979 volume of Les Carnets de l'Enfance, particularly the paper by Emmerij

(29) Emmerij op. cit.

(30) cf Frances Stewart - 1979 - The New International Economic Order and Basic Needs - Nordic Symposium - Development Strategies, Research Policy Institute, University of Lund, Sweden and Singh A - 1979 - The Basic Needs Approach to Development and the NIEO - World Development (June)

(31) Emmerij op. cit. (28)

(32) Nordberg O, Phillips P and Sterky G - 1975 - Action for Children - Towards an Optimum Child Care Package in Africa - Uppsala - Dag Hammarskjöld Foundation

(33) See, for example, the Report on the CICRED/WHO meeting - Geneva - 34 July 1980

(34) WHO/UNICEF - 1979 - Joint WHO/UNICEF Meeting on Infant and Young Child Feeding, Geneva

(35) Chambers R - 1980 - Shortcut Methods in Information Gathering for Rural Development Projects - Institute of Development Studies, Sussex

(36) See Streeten and Hicks op. cit.

(37) See e.g. Ritchie J - 1979 - Learning Better Nutrition - FAO, Rome

(38) See David C. Pitt - 1980 - Open House - WHO/MCH Preliminary Paper

(39) Aarons A and Hawes H - 1979 - Child to Child - London - Macmillan

(40) See ILO - 1980 - Children at Work - Geneva - & Rodgers T and Standing G - 1981 - The Economic Role of Children in Low Income Countries - I.L.O. - Geneva

(41) Chambers R - 1980 - op.cit.

(42) WHO/UNICEF - 1979 - op.cit.

(43) On the weak development in anthropology and sociology of research on the child, see Michelson W. - 1979 -et al. The Child in the City - University of Toronto Press

(44) Some estimates are over 30 million, e.g. the Brandt Report.

(45) Administrative Coordinating Committee of the United Nations System.

CHAPTER ELEVEN

CHANGING NEEDS OF CHILDREN: THE EXPERIENCE OF SRI LANKA*

1. INTRODUCTION

The well-being of children could be regarded as one of the more reliable criteria for evaluating a society's concern for the quality and human content of its development. In terms of this indicator, Sri Lanka's performance ranks relatively high among developing countries. The rapidity with which Sri Lanka has been able to reduce mortality among the young age group and raise their levels of literacy could be considered exceptional for a developing country with a per capita income in the region of 200 US dollars.

These achievements have been an integral part of a process of socio-economic change which from the beginning appears to have accorded a central place to the development of human

*Chapter prepared by Godfrey Gunatilleke, extracted from his paper of the same name pps. 1-2, 15-21, 36, Marga Institute.

resources. The efforts in the field of social development which among other things promoted the well-being of children began during the period of colonial rule, and gathered momentum as the country moved progressively through limited forms of self-government to full independence in the late 1940s. With independence these efforts were further intensified. The provision of basic needs in the form of free health and free education to the population as a whole and the distribution of essential items of food at subsidised or relatively stable prices became the cornerstone of governmental policy for nearly three decades.

Although these efforts fulfilled some of the basic human preconditions for development, it could not be argued that they were conceived as a part of a well formulated strategy for creating the human capital necessary to undertake the major structural changes in Sri Lanka's economy. The failure to transform the economy and expand its productive capacity to match the aspirations that were generated as a result of developments in the social field resulted in the major crisis which overtook the economy from the 1960s onwards, and the social tensions which exploded in the insurrection of 1971. The outlays that had been made in providing for the needs of the age group 0-14 were indeed quite substantial. But these investments were not designed within a framework in which the present needs of this age group were perceived clearly in relation to the longer term future needs and the group moved from the stage of dependence and began to enter the workforce in rapidly increasing numbers. The problems started to surface as the new generation which benefited from the welfare system in the late nineteen-forties and the fifties became the new entrants to the workforce in the mid-sixties. The experience of Sri Lanka therefore underscores the dilemmas which can beset strategies aimed at promoting the well-being of the present population with economic growth and increase of productive capacity to cater to the expanding needs of the future. The change of direction initiated by the present government in Sri Lanka in 1977 was an attempt to bring about a new equilibrium between these conflicting goals, and make fundamental modifications in the policy package which had been adopted in the past. These changes undoubtedly have far-reaching implications for the well-being of the 0-14 age group.

2. THE SYSTEM IN CRISIS

The programmes which promoted the well-being of children were part of a broader programme of social welfare which focused on health, education and food. These elements in the development strategy in Sri Lanka therefore anticipate the more recent approaches which made the satisfaction of basic needs the primary objective of development. Underlying these policies was the acceptance of a benevolent paternalistic role for the state. It was a role conceived within a framework of development values in which the dominant ideology of a Buddhist culture emphasising the importance of 'dhana' (giving and sharing) and 'metta' (compassion) appear to have blended with the concepts of the modern welfare state and made political elites responsive to the need for some degree of equity in the distribution of available resources. But already as the country moved into the sixties the inherent limitations of the system were beginning to manifest themselves and its incapacity to cope with certain deep-seated problems of a structural nature was becoming increasingly evident.

First, the system was encountering a hard core of problems which were not yielding to its efforts. After a rapid drop in infant mortality in the initial phase, the rate of decline below 50 per thousand was proving to be much slower. Having dropped from 82 to 57 in 10 years, it had declined much more slowly to 53.2 in 1965 and 47.5 in 1970, rising again to 51.3 in 1974. The age-specific death rate for the age group 1-4 at approximately 6.2 in 1975 was still excessive for a country which was able to increase average life expectancy to approximately 67. The risk to life in the first seven days of life remained inordinately high. Approximately 42% of infant deaths were occurring during this period, while 60% of infant mortality was in the first month. The evidence available also pointed to a high level of undernourishment for this age group. A survey in 1976 revealed a national average of approximately 6% for acute malnutrition among pre-school children, while chronic malnutrition was as high as 35%. Despite the nation-wide extension of the network of health institutions for child care, the success of the system in reaching the pre-school age group was as yet limited. Where medical technology was capable of achieving results in the short-term and could be applied directly to clearly identified problems of morbidity and prevention of disease as in the case of curative services and immunisation, the system performed fairly effectively and produced visible results. But where it had to deal with more persistent problems which had their origin in poverty, malnutrition, poor sanitation, inadequate knowledge and understanding of health protection and care, the capacity of the system seemed to be as yet very limited.

Second, in the school-going population, despite the availability of free schooling facilities, nearly 15% of the children of school-going age did not enter school at all and on an average another 30% of the children in the age group 5-14 were outside the school system, having dropped out of it at various stages. This segment was therefore not accessible through the formal educational system which is most concerned with the development of this age group. Neither were there non-formal institutions which had developed adequate capacity to deal with specific problems of this group.

Third, and most important of all, the young generation which had been the beneficiaries of this system and moved through it satisfactorily found that they could not get readily integrated into the productive workforce and find useful roles in adult society. The rate of unemployment rocketed to over 20% during this period with the preponderant majority of the unemployed being in the age group 13-24. The high level of unemployment originated from a combination of causes. Clearly, the economy itself had been unable to generate employment at a rate adequate to meet the demand of the growing workforce. At the same time, however, the educational system had promoted job expectations directed at middle-grade non-manual employment expectations which were at variance with the prevailing occupational structure and available job opportunities. Finally, the system had not given adquate attention to the development of technical and vocational skills, as well as attitudes to work which could have better equipped the school leavers for employment.

Fourth, despite the national coverage of the system, significant regional disparities persisted. The most glaring example was the sector comprising the population of Indian descent, resident in the tea plantations. The rural areas surrounding the plantations also appeared to be a seriously disadvantaged segment, with relatively higher rates of infant mortality and malnutrition, and lower rates of school participation. Several districts had social indicators which were far below the national average. In 1974, infant mortality stood at 119 for Nuwara Eliya, 92 for Kandy and 73 for Badulla when the national average was 51. The districts with the lowest rates were Jaffna with 21, Vavuniya and Polonnaruwa with 24, Puttalam with 29 and Moneragala with 31.

Fifth, the prevailing system had fostered dependence on the delivery of services by the State and the provision and administration of servcices had been a top-down process. This was particularly true of services catering to the young age group. This was probably inevitable at the early stages when the State had to assume a benevolent role at a time when levels of education and literacy were relatively low. But the system itself had created a literate population with a much higher capacity for participation than before. It had therefore to make fuller use of the potential for community participation. Elements of community participation which have been present such as the parent-teacher associations, or voluntary organisations such as rural development societies and women's societies were not successful in promoting a self-reliant and self-sustaining process of community participation. Community development programmes have most often been initiatives which have been directed by urban elite groups. The movement had invariably been top-down with hardly any concentration of effort on creating and enhancing the community's own capability for improving health, sanitation, nutrition, and for making full use of the existing potential in the immediate environment for valuable forms of non-formal education.

Sixth, it would be true to say that formal systems administered from the centre, whether they be of health or education, had to an appreciable extent impoverished the capacity at the local level to assume responsibility for forming and developing major facets of children's experience to which the formal systems do not directly address themselves. This applies to the wide range of children's experience in the world of play, in recreation, in the absorption and assimilation of the culture and tradition in society. The traditional sources of nourishment in this area were folk art and culture - whether they be the Jataka stories related by elders, the ceremonies, rites and festivals or other cultural activities such as folk drama. The skills and sources of creativitiy which replenished and sustained them had virtually disappeared from village life. They were also part of a tutelary relationship between elders and young in which culture, tradition and occupational skills were transmitted as a well-integrated process. The modern formal education system effectively disrupted these relationships. Higher levels of literacy and access to new structures of knowledge created a dichotomy between the experience of the young and that of the old. The new system had failed to build up the cultural and extra-curricular counterpart which would have compensated for the disappearance of the traditional forms. This would have required special attention to the recreational, cultural and spiritual needs, to those elements which nurture the creative personality of the child; this would have, among other things, included parks, museums, books, toys, theatre, film, art, broadcasting and TV.

During the period 1965-1977 there were efforts to respond to these deficiencies of the system and to undertake a basic reappraisal of the various components catering to children's needs. New elements were added or existing priorities reordered. The family planning programme began to receive greater attention in the second half of the sixties. In the first half of the seventies a more organised effort in this field was launched and it was included as an important part of the strategy in the Five-Year Plan. Primary health care and preventive services were strengthened in an effort to bring about a better balance between the curative and preventive capacity of the health system. The formation of the Family Health Bureau in 1972,which integrated the maternal and child care services with family planning and health education, provided a more effective institutional framework for co-ordinating activities in this field. A beginning was made during this period to bring nutritional issues to the centre of government policy. Government began to explore systematically the possibility of providing low-cost nutritional supplements. Programmes for health education were also assigned high priority. In the educational system a comprehensive effort was made to restructure the curriculum and to relate it more meaningfully to the world of work and the socio-economic environment giving it a more relevant vocational orientation. These reforms sought to rectify the deficiencies of a system which had contributed to the massive unemployment that emerged in the late sixties and early seventies.

But these readjustments and additions to the health and education systems failed to produce any very significant results. They came during a period when the economy was facing a severe and persistent economic crisis which gathered momentum during the sixties and got intensified in the seventies. The country's terms of trade declined and export earnings lagged far behind the demand for imports. The employment situation continued to deteriorate. Sri Lanka's dependence on imports of food and energy made her specially vulnerable to the world food shortages and the energy crisis in the first half of the seventies. These problems were compounded by the severe droughts which hit the country and the consequent decline in domestic food production during this period. The reduction in the food ration and the resulting hardships were particularly heavy on the disadvantaged groups. This was reflected in the sharp rise in infant mortality from 46.3 in 1973 to 51.3 in 1974. It indicated how susceptible the prevailing conditions were to any external shock or internal crisis which affected the country's import capacity and food supply.

It has to be mentioned however that the mortality rates resumed their downward movement in 1975 and by 1977 had fallen below the lowest death rates reached previously in 1970 (for crude death rate) and 1971 (for infant mortality).

3. THE EIGHTIES

For the decade of the eighties, Sri Lanka should set for itself clearly defined targets in relation to these three main problems.

- The decade should witness a substantial reduction of infant mortality to a rate of approximately 25 per thousand. This would require a considerable improvement of the trends in the seventies.

- By the end of the eighties, the country should have been able to eliminate malnutrition.

- Universal primary education which ensures full school enrolment of the children in the 5-9 age group should be realised before the end of the decade.

It could be argued that the strategies which are being already pursued contain both the programme elements and the institutional framework which would enable us to achieve the targets relating to infant mortality and malnutrition. These include a network of institutions for maternal and child health services capable of reaching the population concerned, the food stamp schemes for poor household in general; programmes for nutritional supplements of malnourished children and mothers, the free midday meal to school children, the activities in the field of primary health and health education. What seems to be needed is not entirely new strategies or new programmes, but rather a more effective strategy of implementation capable of realising the full benefit of the current programmes, with an intensification and strengthening of some of the elements where necessary.

The problems of infant mortality and malnutrition are mainly concentrated in the low income group at the base of the income structure - the bottom 25% which was mentioned earlier. This target group has to be clearly identified in terms of their geographical and sectoral location. The regional variations which have been revealed in socio-economic surveys, surveys of malnutrition and in social indicators such as mortality, give the necessary clues for a much better identification of these target groups. From the data available, the problems themselves are not intractable in size. The segment of high mortality in the 0-30 day period affects approximately 10,000 housholds a year. Rough estimates based on recent surveys of six districts suggest that the proportion of pre-school children suffering from acute malnutrition ranges between 4.6% and 10.2% The number involved could be in the region of 125,000 for the entire island if we assume an average of 7%. The figures also indicate that the chronically undernourished in this group would be approximately 20% or another 300,000 children. If we assume that the proportion of anaemic mothers had not changed significantly from 1976, the year of the malnutrition survey carried out by CARE, the number of anaemic mothers needing special nutritional supplement and care would be approximately 125,000. The proportion of malnourished children increases as we move to the older age cohorts in the 5-9 age group and beyond, rising to an average of about 40%. This would amount to another 650,000 children in the 5-9 age group. This means that any plan of action aimed at dealing effectively with the problem of malnutrition should have the capacity to reach a little over a million children.

The eradication of malnutrition in the long-term depends on the success with which the development strategy in the eighties raises the poverty group to levels at which basic needs are adequately fulfilled. Until then programmes of state intervention and income support would have to be implemented effectively for the benefit of the disadvantaged groups. The existing programmes have to be assessed first for their capacity to cater to the entire group which is affected, second for the adequacy of the support already given in order to make a significant impact on malnutrition, and third, for the integrity of the system in transferring the benefits of the scheme in full to the intended beneficiaries. On all these criteria the existing system appears to be inadequate. In regard to the food stamp scheme, the issues that have been raised earlier, such as the impact of inflation on the value of food stamps become relevant. The estimates of the present coverage of the state intervention programmes for children and mothers, indicate that probably not more than 2/3rds of the malnourished children in the pre-school group and undernourished mothers are reached. The per capita supply as well as its regularity do not appear to have reached the required standards. The programme has not taken adequate account of regional disparities. Finally, abuses in the distribution systems are also present. To eliminate these abuses it would be necessary to mobilise much greater participation by the community in the management and monitoring of these services.

Part of the problem of malnutrition in the age group above five could be dealt with effectively through the school system with an improved school medical service and the scheme for midday meals. This would still leave out the large proportion of children who are outside the school system. In the long-term, the problem could be partly solved if universal free education is achieved by the end of the decade. But until then, special measures are required if the malnourished segment in the 5-9 age group is to receive care and attention. There is no programme at present specifically directed at the physical well-being of this segment.

The problems relating to children of school-going age who are out of the school system have received little or no attention. These children are not easily reached through any existing institutional machinery. The programme specific to this group of children would have to be developed on two fronts. First, it would be necessary to pay more concentrated attention to the problems of drop-outs, examine the social and economic causes for this phenomenon, and through existing institutions such as the parent-teacher associations and other community organisations, assist in the process of preventing drop-outs, and where drop-outs occur, speedily bringing them back to the system. Apart from measures designed to increase the rate of retention in the system, it would also be necessary to provide programmes of non-formal education to children in this age group who are out of the school system. While there are no easy answers to this problem it has to be pointed out that there has been no attempt to deal specifically with the needs of this group. Any strategy for the welfare of children cannot afford to neglect this group.

Besides the short and medium-term programmes relating to the urgent problems of children's welfare, any serious national effort at planning for children would need to formulate a long-term perspective which deals with the changing needs of children during the next two decades, particularly in relation to the demographic as well as economic changes which have been indicated in the development scenario that is likely to unfold. In such a long-term perspective, the hitherto neglected aspects of children's well-being would have to receive greater attention. With reduced demand for quantitative expansion there would be greater scope for the allocation of resources for qualitative improvement. If the same proportion of national income as is spent at present continues to be spent on the child population, the planners would have to examine how the additional resources that would be available with the rise in national income could be spent on improving the quality of life of children over the next two decades.

The resources that would become available would have to be estimated in broad magnitudes and the areas of priority in regard to qualitative improvements would need to be identified. These could include the provision of a wide range of community goods, such as parks, recreation services, museums and libraries which pay special attention to children's needs, and children's resorts. The child's world outside the school would have to be enriched in addition to the enrichment of the life in school. Facilities for the care and socialisation of the pre-school child will be required to cater to the new needs that will arise with increasing participation of women in the workforce. More resources could be allocated to strengthen and expand school health services and improve the midday meal. The entire field of children's literature, media, and the arts would require much more systematic planning and promotion than there have been in the past. A long-term perspective on the world of the child as we move into the nineties and approach the turn of the century will have to take account of these possibilities and plan to cater to the changing pattern of needs.

4. DEVELOPMENT VALUES AND GOALS RELATING TO CHILDREN

The place of the child in the development strategies of developing countries would be determined by the character of the strategy that is being pursued, its central objectives and goals, and the principal means adopted to achieve them. A strategy which is highly growth-oriented and which is primarily dependent on the market both for its productive sectors as well as its services, will affect the well-being of children in a way which is significantly different from the way in which an equity-oriented strategy with a bias towards social welfare and the satisfaction of children's needs for their present well-being would do. In the former, children are essentially conceived as resources and assets, as a future factor of production which has to be developed with care and attention. In the latter, the accent would fall more clearly on the improvement of present well-being and the alleviation of present deprivation. Both approaches have their own intrinsic concern for the well-being of children, each with a different emphasis in the development values which guide it.

Sri Lanka's own efforts at promoting the well-being of children has been guided more by the social-welfare approach directed at improvement of the conditions of the specific age group rather than by a manpower-planning or resource development objective. In the provision of free health, free education, and distribution of subsidised food rations, it removed the main cluster of basic needs of children from the market economy of exchange and made it a part of the grant economy,the economy of public welfare. Implicit in the removal was a framework of non-economic values which set the parameters for the policies and development strategies of the government. While these values derived partly from the concepts of the modern welfare state, they were easily accommodated within and were reinforced by the traditional Buddhist value system. The size and character of the "grant" economy is an indicator of the quality of life in a society, its capacity at sharing, at enjoyment in community. It becomes particularly important for the well-being of the dependent population - children and old people. Therefore, in the post '77 effort to find a new equilibrium between equity and growth, between present well-being and needs of the future, it is essential to preserve the ethical core which guided the process of social development in the past.

All societies, whether traditional or modern, will see in their children the image of the future society. In the traditional society, with its very slow pace of socio-economic change and relatively stable value system, the "manpower" planning was essentially a slow initiation and preparation of children for adult roles which themselves changed little over time. As a result the passage from childhood to adulthood was an integrated process in which the sharp discontinuities were managed within a complex system of values and beliefs. The world of play, the apprenticeship to adults both in the workplace and household, the rites and ceremonies which marked the challenge of moving from childhood to adulthood was one unified experience of growing up, in which the relationship between the generations was relatively free of conflict, and the values governing the relationship stressed the intrinsic meaning and worth of each stage of life from childhood to old age. Within this framework of values the patterns of upbringing to condition the child for his future adult role and impart the necessary values and skills for fulfilling this role were in equilibrium with the concern for the enjoyment of his childhood as a stage of life. This of course is an ideal representation of the value-orientation in traditional societies. Acute scarcity of resources often took its toll of human life and within the normal priorities of survival it tended to discriminate against the youngest segment of the population. Parental love and all the primal bonds relating to reproduction and nurture of the young had at times to yield to inescapable problems of balancing population and resources. In such a situation the needs of the dependent population came after those of the active and productive workforce. Hence the incidence of infanticide in some of the traditional societies.

The process of modernisation has released forces which have radically disturbed this traditional equilibrium which had both positive and negative features. First, modernisation implied a process of change. This signified a period of preparation in the childhood for adult roles which were very different from the roles of the parental generation. It was therefore a process of preparation in which the parental relationship could play only a very limited function. It consequently separated the parental roles from the functions of learning and initation into adult society. It thereby brought a serious cleavage between the formation of values for the totality of living, the conduct of interpersonal relationships in family and society on the one hand, and the acquisition of skills and knowledge for modern occupations on the other. These disruptions and discontinuities were seldom taken into account in the formal preparation of the young in the process of modernisation. Apart from these disruptive effects which were to some extent an inevitable part of modernisation and structural change, the objectives for the preparation of the young were essentially oriented towards technological and economic growth. The framework for the development of children was ideally one which became part of an overall exercise in mapower planning which had as its terminal objective the satisfaction of the manpower needs of the economy.

The preparation of children in terms of future roles is as we saw part of any society. The "manpower planning" approach is in this primary sense integral to the functioning of any society. The purposive link between the present life of the child and his future roles is essential, it is the way in which future prospects are perceived and integrated into the world of play and learning that surrounds childhood with a sense of security and meaning about the future. In this sense even the toys, the games and children's mythology form the values of children and prepare children for their later roles. For example, the world of play around "cowboys and Indians" or the institution of scouting had its relevance for the child and its upbringing in the migrant European settlements in the North American continent at one stage of its history. The neglect of the linkages between the present well-being of childhood and the demands of future adulthood can lead to a situation in which a relatively healthy literate generation of children will in time enter an adult society which is not organised to receive them -a situation which is partly reflected in the Sri Lankan crisis in the early seventies.

But the approach to the child through concepts of modern manpower planning can be narrowly functional in focus. Children's well-being then becomes conceptualised mainly in terms of economic rationality. It serves its purpose mainly in terms of future efficiency as a manpower input into the system. In such an approach many aspects of upbringing and nurture could be ignored. It is likely to fail to project childhood as a stage of life which has to be experienced and enjoyed in all its richness. Its bias will be to develop the child for its future economic and technical roles without adequate attention to its spiritual nourishment, the formation of values, and the accumulation of the knowledge and wisdom to cope with and respond to human experience as a whole.

To conceive of childhood in a "holistic framework" is to approach it with developmental values which are significantly different from those which inform a strategy based on narrow manpower-planning concepts. In such an approach the concern to enrich the experience of the child materially and spiritually, to identify and satisfy the needs specific to childhood would be balanced and integrated with the concern to prepare him or her for future roles and functions. The home with its environment of love, affection and primal bonds, the social institutions for health care and physical well-being, the world of learning, the world of recreation and play, the links to the religious institutions and centres of spiritual nourishment must each receive its due place in a strategy aimed at enhancing the quality of life for children. The assumptions that are made in a strategy of this kind have far-reaching implications for the upbringing of children and their preparation for adult life.

There is recognition, here, that the extent of fulfilment in childhood and the unfolding of experience at this stage have a significant bearing on the patterns of adult behaviour and the health and sanity of the entire social system. It is acknowledged that the material and spiritual deprivation that may occur at this stage of life can find expression in the deformities and social neuroses of adult society. Recent writing draws attention, for instance, to the adverse effects which the intense competitiveness of the modern examination system and the profound insecurity it breeds is tending to have on social organisations as a whole. Perceptions of this nature call for a greater awareness and understanding of children's needs and better integration of child-specific programmes and policies in the national development strategy than has been done hitherto. These problems are compounded in a developing society where the needs of the young have to be dealt with in the transition from a predominantly agrarian society to the technological order. Development planners have given little attention to these aspects, particularly the fundamental tensions and conflicts that are generated in the inner world of the child and adolescent. It would seem that development planning for children would need much greater intellectual and analytical inputs to these aspects than are at present available.

The implementation of such a strategy requires a basic reorientation of the centrally organised top-down planning and delivery of services which has been hitherto characteristic of Sri Lanka's welfare system. It has to emphasise the role of the community and its participation. The parental generation and the community in general have to be incorporated as partners in child development and the roles they traditionally performed recast and given new responsibility and meaning in the modern setting. This becomes all the more important in the light of the governments effort to create a decentralised institutional framework in which village development councils will play a role. Concern for the well-being of children could become a prime mover. It can mobilise community participation for the entire development effort which moves upward from the village level, over a whole range of activities ranging from agricultural activities for nutritional self-reliance to pre-school programmes of child care, and public goods such as places of recreation, children's parks, libraries, and centres of cultural and creative activitiy for children. The present welfare programmes for children as pointed out earlier has concentrated on a few basic needs; it has largely neglected the range of recreational, cultural and spiritual needs and the development of the creative personality of children. More active participation of the parents and the community could help in a much more diversified extra-curricular life for the school-going population as well as a richer socialisation process for the pre-school children. It would also be much more effective in dealing with the persistent problems of morbidity and mortality in the most vulnerable infant groups where the hazards are largely in the home and the immediate community environment and where the upgrading of care by parents is of the first importance. The entire effort to enhance the quality of life of the pre-school group depends largely on the parents and the local community, as is being demonstrated in some of the programmes in primary health care and in the Sarvodaya efforts.

The child-specific development effort which links the stage of childhood to the adult roles by the holistic nature of its concern for human needs will need to go beyond the needs of manpower planning. It will have to be concerned as much with the formation of values and with the aquisition of occupational skills and scientific knowledge. The preparation of the young in Sri Lanka would therefore have to address itself to the problem areas in Sri Lanka's pluralistic society. From the very early processes of socialisation the inculcation of values and habits of thoughts must contribute towards the gro of a conflict-free multi-ethnic society. This means that in the early stages of developing the child's outlook, forms of play, both the oral and written tradition for children, the perception of history, the appreciation of the fine arts and crafts, must promote the environment for such a society. This is indeed a very demanding task as it requires the development of a whole system of communication through the period of schooling, higher learning and the rest of society which lays the basis of values, perceptions, and concepts which work in favour of national harmony, and remove inherited communalistic biases and prejudices. Similarly, the value-formation in childhood has to lay the groundwork for adult roles and the disciplines required in a modern society. These include the work-ethic essential for development, the nature of civic participation and responsbility needed for the efficient functioning of a free democratic society, the capacity for tolerance, communication and interchange in a society in which dissent, opposition and civic freedoms are fundamental to the system. It is important in this connection to note that the formation of values in the young generation plays a primary role in the socialist countries. This of course would be criticised as ideological conditioning, but regardless of the controversial issues in the particular mode of value-formation adopted in these societies, basic elements of the process are those of harmoniously integrating the young in adult society. Any society needs to have the equivalent of this process adapted to its own social goals and ideology.

The issues that have been discussed stress the central importance of the child-specific component of any development strategy. It is certainly a component which cannot be dealt with in disparate parts which are dispersed in a fragmented way in different parts of the system. It requires strategic guidance from a central point in the system which is capable of integrating the different aspects ranging from what might be described as the enriching "stage of life" approach to the manpower planning and preparation for adult roles in a consistent complementary whole. In Sri Lanka the cluster of child-oriented activities which have been brought together under the Ministry of Plan Implementation provides a beginning for such strategic planning for the well-being of children.

CHAPTER TWELVE

FUTURE ACTION RESEARCH NEEDS - THE CASE OF THE SOUTH PACIFIC*

One must begin by noting that as yet no significant research has been done where the skills of the medical practitioner and the social scientist have been combined to examine the social aspects of child health in the South Pacific. But this is not to deny that those with medical qualifications have worked assiduously on important aspects of health to achieve significant improvements in the South Pacific. Equally social scientists in a variety of disciplines, either together or singly, and largely in the context of their own discipline rather than utilising a multi-disciplinary methodology, have produced their tomes for doctoral theses or publications. The two groups have worked frequently in isolation with some awareness of one another's work but with little or no cooperation or even interaction. This paper attempts to postulate some ways in which this gap might be bridged by bringing the medical practitioners and social scientists together. Since basic work is required one

*Paper prepared by Ahmed Ali

might suggest that the Pacific in this research area remains a virgin field to be ploughed in cooperation. Thus an opportunity also exists for experiments in the use of new methodologies and perhaps the formulation of new theories. This paper itself is an exploration, what it recommends is not in any way definitive. It is written from the point of view of a social scientist with the hope of enabling comments from others in the same field as well as medical doctors with the hope that out of the discussion and the criticism will emerge something which will permit action-oriented research in the future aimed at improving human welfare.

The islands of the South Pacific lie scattered over thousands of square kilometers of ocean with considerable distance between countries. They exhibit not only a variety in their physical characteristics but also in the cultures of their people. There is considerable difference between the atolls of Kiribati and Tuvalu and the volcanic islands of Melanesia. Some of the diversity is captured in the traditional categorization of Melanesia, Polynesia and Micronesia. No less evident are the differences found in their distinct approach to life and the social structure and political organization ranging from the conservative kingdom of Tonga to the more democratic islands to its west among them the multi-racial and multi-cultural state of Fiji and the multi-lingual islands of Vanuatu and the Solomons. There are nevertheless some common features too. They are all islands; they are small; they are all developing countries; some are even classified among the least developed nations of the world. Apart from the nickel in New Caledonia and deposits of copper in Namosi in Fiji and gold in Vatukoula in Fiji, the phosphate of Nauru and the Ocean Islands, there is an absence of natural resources. There is no oil despite continuing prospecting for it. There are no major industries if the sugar industry of Fiji is left aside. At the same time the islands lack some of the hectic pace of life that is found in the industrial countries of the developed world. The people are largely rural dwelling, practising agriculture, either commercial or subsistence. Many rely on the soils to provide them with food supplemented by what is found in the sea around them. The casual visitor normally notes the pleasantness of the sunshine and the comfort of the beaches with some awareness of the hungry sharks beyond them. Though there is poverty and an absence of wealth for the majority, one fails to find the abject destitution and the misery that one encounters in parts of Asia. A quick general impression is that there are no major problems of health in these islands yet what is seen on the surface should not be allowed to mistake myth for reality. A recent committee investigating health in Fiji came to the conclusion: "the standard of health of the people of Fiji is generally good" It went on to add:

> The main areas of concern which will require close monitoring by the Ministry of Health in the coming years are the problems of nutrition affecting young children and mothers in pregnancy and the accompanying complications of anaemia in pregnant mothers giving rise to babies of low birth weight, a high infant mortality and increased predisposition to maternal mortality; the mosquito borne diseases such as filariasis, dengue haemorrhagic fever and measles and the increasing incidents of sexually transmitted diseases and road transport accidents (1).

For the coral atoll to the north, Kiribati, the Pacific Islands Year Book noted "diarrhoeal disease is very common and can only be reduced as safe water supplies and better waste disposal are provided"(2). It went on to point out that in 1977 eighteen deaths resulted from cholera. Again emphasising the need for stricter measures regarding water control and sanitation the Handbook of the Solomon Islands admitted that the chief epidemic diseases continued to be malaria and tuberculosis. It added "gastroenteritis, occurring in localised epidemics, is a big problem in young children (usually arising from contaminated water supplies)" (3). These examples would suffice to suggest that health remains a major source of anxiety for the countries of the South Pacific.

Since our concern lies with the young it would be worthwhile noting that in the case of Fiji 41% of its population was under the age of 15 at the time of the last census in 1976. For Cook Islands, 50% are in this category and in American Samoa 45%, whereas in Tonga a country which is bedevilled by rapidly rising population confronted with limited availability of land, 41% of its people are under the age of 16 years. In this situation the first piece of work that might be done would be a general study for each country on health and development. A broad picture outlining the characteristics of health and development in each Pacific Island state is important to enable comparability among them. Such studies might as a result of the comparisons,establish certain common features or they may highlight special characteristics in important aspects and could suggest the next step in solution-seeking research. These studies would take as given, the concept of basic needs for development, the idea of primary health care, which for instance is emphasised in Fiji's latest Development Plan and also accept the possibility of health for all by the year 2000.

Our task, however, is to find how relationships may be established between health and other aspects of life in order to improve the quality of life for all. In the case of the Pacific, as perhaps anywhere else, we might begin by examining what we might call the traditional practices of child rearing. This is important because many of the developing countries have been subjected to tradition-destroying colonial rule and have only recently become independent. In the process of foreign domination, through advice and forced change, in many cases they have had to relinquish what they had developed themselves over the ages when they were free. Many were convinced or coerced into accepting that what they had was no longer of value or of use and hence they had to give way to what was described as modern. The same process often persuaded them that they ought to use for their children commercially prepared food in attractive tins produced in some western industrialized country. It is therefore not surprising to learn that in Fiji breast-feeding has declined as is also the case in many other parts of the Pacific. This has come about not only through the propaganda that was originally brought in the colonial period and persisted subsequently but it is also the consequence of both parents having to earn a living in order to maintain the standard of living that they have got used to. It is therefore considerably more convenient to buy pre-packaged and already prepared food and milk. The change in the direction toward the original methods will only come about through concerted efforts towards decolonizing the mind.

By going back and producing studies of practices in earlier periods and seeing how these practices affected child health it is very easy to conclude that since colonial rule and missionary advice put an end to endemic diseases and introduced new medicine everything else that they offered was equally invaluable while all things indigenous utilised before their advent were of no purpose or in fact detrimental to health. A study of traditional medicine thus becomes essential. Indeed this is necessary, not only because traditional medicine might be cheaper, but it may also indicate how some of the traditional herbs were more effective than the anti-biotics that one has to buy at exhorbitant prices from the pharmacist downtown. While some work has already got underway in the Pacific in these two areas, there is need to quicken the tempo, particularly in evaluating the role of traditional medicine and earlier traditional child-rearing practices for life in today's world. To advocate this is not to call for a total debunking of western medicine or of new scientific practices, rather there is a need to assess the two together because tradition and modernity are not always necessarily in conflict. Problems have arisen where one has been emphasised at the expense of the other. If on the other hand tradition and modernity were seen complementing each other then the effectiveness of both would have been enhanced and perhaps in the long term the health of the community might have improved rather than have been subjected to a process where at one stage one was fashionable and at another the other acquired permanence or was resorted to surreptitiously. Any reassessment must have implications for the educational systems of the South Pacific. It would mean making these systems more functional and relevant to the needs they must satisfy. Purely formal education for its own sake is not necessarily going to be effective.

In a recent study based on Ethopia, Dr. Nebiat Tafari pointed out that "formal education had surprisingly no significant effect on the timely use of antenatal services" (4). The lesson in this for us is that merely by teaching issues relating to health and development or studying them in the curricula of the school, either at secondary level or at universities at the tertiary level, changes will not automatically emerge. What we must concentrate on is functional education. For instance, what would be necessary would be a programme to convince mothers as well as the young of the value of re-examining and re-accepting what was traditional. Some lessons might be taken from the effectiveness of the selling of family planning in the Pacific. Success did not have much to do with the literacy rate of the people. It was accepted because it was regarded as pragmatic in that if one had too many children one could not go to work or one could not acquire certain other material benefits or indeed not be able to cater for them adequately. The posters which are found on the walls of health clinics and other public places in both rural areas and urban centres, pointing out the advantages of a small family, could very well be copied and with similar slogans to provide health education. One might remember the Chinese adage that one good picture is worth a thousand words. In attempting such a programme one would have to ascertain what are the most effective ways of communicating in South Pacific cultures. Who are the most trusted givers of messages, what are the most effective means of conveying lessons. It would entail finding out whether in fact the current methods of sending messages are effective and practicable. Is the modern doctor in some ways as convincing as the missionary of the nineteenth century, if not, why not? To begin with, is the gospel of the new discoveries getting through to those who have most need of knowing the results? Are pregnant mothers in rural areas, for example, being told of the importance of feeding their babies themselves, of the changes that are taking place not only in their own body, but also of the unborn whom they are carrying; do they know or have they forgotten the traditional foods which gave strength to their predecessors?

This perhaps brings us to the whole question of how health is planned for a community. If it is all done by the Ministry of Health based in the capital city, which then conveys its views to the planning commission or the department of planning, which then adds its prejudices, or goes through with a red pencil, through what the health element has recommended for budgetary reasons of inadequate finance, then it is very unlikely that the health programme, which has been debated and approved in Parliament or some other august national body, without any grassroots consultation, - it is unlikely to succeed in toto. It becomes yet one more plan or programme imposed from above, not fully understood by the people, no matter how well intentioned it is, no matter how useful its long term results might prove to be if it is implemented. Hence in evaluating any health programme one should begin by enquiring how it was planned, who contributed to the various ingredients in it. Only then should one attempt to assess the delivery system. To suggest that there must be widespread participation or involvement of people in determining what is in their best interests in terms of health is not merely to subscribe to the latest fashion about participatory democracy. If people do not have a say in what they are expected to execute then it is very unlikely that they would welcome innovation in a whole-hearted manner especially, if what they are being required to accept conflicts with habits long-established, no matter how bad or retrogressive these may be from the point of view of those well-versed in modern medicine, and who know what is best for the health of community. Ordinary people might find prescriptions provided from the outside irksome and may in fact see those who write them as extremely arrogant if they have not had a chance to communicate their own views or to make their own suggestions. To recommend involvement or participation is not to advocate that all that is given from below must be incorporated automatically into a national plan. Indeed in the exchange and interaction that will take place those who know most about medicine may through dialogue be able to convince ordinary villagers or urban dwellers in squatter surroundings as to what is in their best interest. And in the process those in decision-making may also learn how they may be best able to get their message home through cooperation instead of having to impose their policies when encountering resistance.

Planning has to be decentralized in order to neutralise the ill-effects of centralization. Here too one has to look at the communication processes in a community in order to discover how the two-way flow of messages occurs. One needs to find out from rural villagers and urban dwellers on the outskirts of the city as well as those on the fringes of society, about the practices they have hitherto used and the effectiveness of these. One may need to explain laboriously issues about health to ordinary people before deciding what is best for them. Since disadvantaged groups often blame their Government as the source of all their ills and come to regard authority as something irksome and always operating against them, they consider themselves helpless and become indifferent and even antagonistic towards what they see as yet another directive from their oppressor. While in the Pacific overtly authority is respected there are subtle ways of disregarding its injunctions. In traditional societies in a situation of change authority is frequently respected for ceremonial purposes and occasions while at the same time it is undergoing transformation and its strength is being eroded. One needs to note such realities and evaluate their influence for delivering health systems.

Pacific Island leaders have frequently voiced their doubts about the effectiveness of governmental and administrative structures which they have inherited from colonial rulers. They seem concerned that they are not able to communicate adequately and accurately with their own people. Many of them seem to think that they were able to get their messages across much more quickly, much more effectively, through their own traditional methods. They have called for a re-examination of these as well as a study of alternative forms of government and administration to cater for the needs of small societies which are proud of their traditional heritage. Not only must we concern ourselves with a relevant health system but we need to explore whether we have an appropriate administrative system to deliver it, for the South Pacific island states there is no study available which has examined this crucial relationship. There is an urgent need for research in this aspect of government as it affects health programmes..

There is also the need to investigate ways in which the relationship between health and what has been called social welfare might be improved. If we use the example of Fiji's Eigth Development Plan and note what it has to say about social welfare we would quickly find that the recipients are people whose health in one way or another is also endangered or affected. The Plan says:

> The objective is to provide aid through cash or kind to members of the community who without such support would suffer severe deprivation. Four main groups in the community fall into this category:
> a) children without proper parental care;
> b) destitute families;
> c) the aged; and
> d) those with severe mental or physical disabilities(5).

Indeed those who qualify for social welfare benefits find that often their position is discovered as a consequence of the adverse state of their health. Second, if for its part social welfare is to play a preventive role it must discover those who are in need of social welfare assistance before their physical or mental condition deteriorates to a level where they have no need of the physician. The two departments, of Health and Social Welfare, must work together.

In a study that the present author has been carrying out on the Social Welfare and Development Policy of Fiji he found that many of the traditional ways of dealing with those in need of social welfare were disappearing because of changes not only as a result of the arrival of the monetarized economy but also because of the movement of many people away from villages into towns. This necessitated more frequent intervention on the part of the state to fill the vacuum created by the transformation which society was undergoing. Social welfare workers in various parts of Viti Levu also pointed out that there was an increasing incidence of breakdown in Indian marriages. There was also an increase in the number of children born out of wedlock, both amongst Indians and Fijians. Secondly, it was pointed out that unmarried mothers amongst Indians were often turned away from their homes and not re-accepted until they had found an adoptive parent for their child. While in the Fijian situation often the existing social structure found some way of absorbing the child born out of wedlock, in the Indian system the family because of the fear of loss of face would only in very rare and indeed exceptional circumstances accept such a child. Not only was the child likely to be affected in such situations, the mother from the stage of pregnancy and even beyond was under considerable stress and strain.

Further, there was also an increasing reluctance on the part of many families to care for their aged. There was greater attempt to rely upon the assistance of an Old People's Home. These new appraches to old problems reflect a change in the value system. While the examples here are drawn from Fiji, there is some indication that these changes may also be evident in other parts of the Pacific. The area of Social Welfare has a bearing on family life and issues affecting the family have ramifications for the young as well as the old. It is not only the parents who are affected but also their progeny, whether they be under five or under twenty-one. There seem to have been few, if any, recent studies on family life in the Pacific, particularly in the way it is changing amidst a barrage of factors, not only from the outside but also as a result of occurrences in the country itself, or indeed within a particular society itself as it adjusts to new situations and new needs and new aspirations of its members. Recently in a paper titled "The Health and Welfare of Fourth World Families: Issues and Policies for the Future', Professor Jerzy Zubrzycki suggested the need for the planning of parent-centred programmes in health and education. He contended: "To effect a change in the conditions of health of fourth world children requires solidarity with their families"(6).

This advice could be applied to the South Pacific in its present stage of development. Traditionally the family has been the linchpin in the advancement of a group in the South Pacific but evidence shows that due to a number of socio-economic factors the role of the family is altering. We do not know to what extent this revision in the role of the family is causing a number of stresses. We are told that the extended family system is on the decline and with it is disappearing an institution which provided some cushioning effect for its members in times of stress. We need to find out whether the state can now take up the functions previously performed by the extended family system or whether new devices have to be found or indeed whether one ought to make concerted efforts to buttress the family system and to strengthen the extended system itself. While such a comment might appear retrogressive or obscurantist in some societies, it may not be so for the South Pacific where people are still deeply attached to strong kinship ties which they feel are essential for the survival of indigenous social structure and with it their cultures. One is inclined to contend that a blow is being delivered to the family as a social unit through outward migration and urbanization plus other factors.

The problems of the family cannot be dissociated from the difficulties encountered by youth in the Pacific. When one visits the towns of the various island states one finds more and more young people standing around apparently with little to do. This may be more evident in Suva than Honiara for instance or even Vila but Honiara and Vila are as afflicted with growing unemployment as Suva is. Given their limited resources, their small economies, it is very unlikely that the Pacific Islands will be able to generate the number of jobs required to gainfully employ all the school leavers. A study by A.H. Wood and Elizabeth Wood Ellem on Tonga stated "Overcrowding in the main town, unemployment and increased crime (especially among adolescents) are consequences of the population explosion and shortage of land"(7).

A businessman from Vanuatu wrote in cautious terms of his own country "Our population is growing at a rapid rate, getting younger and more demanding through education. The rural sector can absorb unemployment but life in the outer islands must be made more attractive"(8). These words hardly reflect optimism. And another Vanuatuan writing on the economy of his country said "The government's own resources for capital development are small if not non-existent ... and we will rely heavily at least for the next 5 to 7 years, on aid from donor countries to implement the proposed development plan, and Vanuatu will not be able to meet her recurrent budget either for the next 5 years"(9).

The report of the Financial Review Committee in Fiji was even more gloomy in its comments: "We estimate that between 1976 and 1991, over 118,000 new jobs will need to be created to employ all new entries to the labour force and absorb existing employment. This is nearly 8,000 additional jobs a year --- a number equivalent to all teachers or all construction workers now employed, or 51 new Carlton Breweries each year"(10). When the young remain unemployed and idle they find their own means to occupy their time. These are often ways and means which deviate from norms that society has laid down for its own stability and continuity. We know that crime frequently accompanies unemployment but we are frequently reluctant to accept that the unemployed often go without meals or even resort to alcohol and when they cannot purchase alcoholic beverages in order to find solace and escape from misery in them they manufacture their own commodities using such harmful liquids as methylated spirits to satisfy their needs. Many of these young men in the Pacific who will be unemployed or are unemployed are not drop-outs from school, they have successfully completed their secondary level education in many cases and some will have completed their studies at tertiary institutions. The unemployed in the future will include young people with ability who are frustrated and will regard as the cause of their discontent the prevailing socio-economic system and the existing power structure --- their anger will have implications not only for law and order but for existing institutions which uphold status quo.

Unemployment is likely to be largely a urban phenomenon as people move into towns, looking for jobs but being unable to find them. But those who remain in the rural areas will languish in the subsistence sector and will be largely under-employed; they too will not be able to earn enough to satisfy their basic needs. There might be peace in the rural sector but it is likely that the urban unemployed may disaffect them too and draw them into their network in an alliance of all dissident elements in the nation. Among these could very well be the squatters whose colonies seem to be proliferating on the outskirts of many towns in the Pacific. These squatters everywhere have one common characteristic in that they do not have land of their own and are domiciled on what belongs to someone else; they are aware of this predicament of theirs and remain forever insecure. A recent study of the squatter colony outside Ba, a town in north-west Viti Levu in Fiji, indicated that the squatters were suffering from ill health and their condition was likely to deteriorate further and with rapidity.

A welfare organisation in Suva reported that poverty was on the rise generally. In its report it contended that many poor mothers were unable to breast feed their babies possibly because of their own diet. It added that a mother's short stay in a maternity clinic did not allow her time for the breast milk to begin flowing and for her to learn how to breast feed. It also found that there was a decline in the earlier enthusiasm for promoting family planning in Fiji. It suspected that many marital difficulties were the result of inflation and money problems. The organization warned women against de facto relationships because it had found that men in the low income group were unable to support their legal family and had deserted them and were doing likewise to women with whom they developed a subsequent liaison. It also advised women that their extended family group was no longer able to come to the rescue: at the most it would help perhaps for a week or two but then its assistance declined and ceased. One could not expect much help in a situation where $38 in 1970 had the same purchasing power as $100 in 1980 and this had affected the poorer segments very severely.

Many of the people the organisation had to deal with were persons who were living in a rented room in a town or in a squatter settlement where they had no gardens to plant their own food.

In the light of such comments from social welfare organizations close to the poor it is essential that the relationship between poverty and urban settlements in the Pacific needs urgent study. The incidence of poverty has been ignored amidst the propaganda of travel brochures about happy contented natives with smiling faces, or even scholarly works through remarks such as those of E.K. Fisk about subsistence affluence(11). Such tales tend to remind one of the view of the European settlers in the nineteenth century: they always believed dogmatically that the natives always had too much and should relinquish their land for economic development through the private enterprise of the white men. While it is true that in the South Pacific one does not encounter the destitution and open misery evident in parts of Asia it does not mean that there is no poverty in the Pacific. Poverty in a country has to be measured against what is available to the different groups in a community, different classes if you wish.

The poor of the Pacific are those without adequate land, those without employment, those without adequate opportunities to educate their children, in other words those who are unable to satisfy the very basic needs of food and shelter by being unable to earn a reasonable livelihood. There is no doubt that many of these would be the urban squatters or the unemployed in the towns, but there are also some who continue to live in the rural areas and are unemployed or underemployed and though they may be able to grow some of their requirements they cannot obtain all they need because they live in an economy where money is essential to purchase some basic commodities. Such inequality and deprivation leads among other things to an unbalanced diet and poor health.

The issue of poverty as it relates to health should be looked at then in the context of both rural development as well as urbanisation. The relationship between poverty, rural existence, and health deserves examination because the majority of Pacific Islanders despite their migration to urban areas continue to dwell in the rural sector. Such a study should be linked to another which investigates how those who have left the rural world for the towns are faring in health terms especially as increasingly this movement out from the rural part is not circular migration but is consistently becoming a permanent exodus into urban life.

The answer to these problems does not lie simply in economic development meaning growth. To illustrate some of the difficulties one might use the example of tourism in the Pacific. While tourism seems to have brought some monetary or economic benefits, with it have also come a number of social evils. It might help strengthen foreign exchange by bringing profits to those who own hotels or duty-free shops, it may provide employment for some as well but these can be accompanied by deleterious effects. For instance, those employed in the urban areas in tourist services may have to leave their village and family behind, thus causing strain and strife in the family structure. Those working in hotels, close to the bar may be inclined to imbibe more than they would have otherwise. In a study of the effect of tourism in Western Samoa, Malama and Penelope Meleisea have pointed out that resources required for village water supply might be utilised in Apia in the interest of the tourist industry despite the need being more urgent in the rural sector. They argue that with a concentration of finance for development in the urban sector the rural area tends to be neglected and many villages are liable to suffer severe water shortages. Besides, the concentration of industrial development on hotels creates competition between industrial needs and those of the local people. Further delicacies such as crab and crayfish and certain fruits become priced beyond the ability of locals and find their way to the hotels to feed tourists(12). Paula Nikula writing about the impact of tourism on the village of Suvavou, near the capital city of Fiji, contends that there are significant social costs. Wives selling handicrafts do not arrive home in time to cook meals for their husbands and use their work in Suva as an excuse to avoid domestic duties. Consequently, there is tension between husband and wife and children are neglected. Some children because of neglect even fail to go to school and in Nikula's view become a nuisance to passing visitors on the road. Tension also arises between parents and young people who are attracted in the evenings to the hotel where tourist entertainment occurs. He adds, "new styles of dress and late night dances worry parents, especially when they result in unwanted pregnancies and trouble with the police"(13). In their study of tourism in Kiribati, Peter Tong and Beingham Tanentoa, suggest that there are adverse implications for the natural environment through tourism and its accompanying phenomenon of urbanization. They state:

> One effect has been the removal of coconut trees and other vegetation to make room for more buildings. This is giving rise to a considerbale amount of soil erosion which causes sedimentation, harming the shallow water marine communities surrounding the coastal line. Luxurious mangroves, sea grass and coral flats that once surrounded the lagoon coastline are now declining, and with them the fish catches also decline(14).

> Another effect of urbanization on Tarawa is caused by poor sewerage. Pit latrines and over the water toilets are familiar sites, but the accumulation of wastes under these buildings leads to the widespread polution of inshore waters, making fish and selfish unfit for consumption, making swimming dangerous both for local residents and tourists alike. In fact, it was held responsible for the outbreak of cholera in 1977.
>
> Urbanization also increases the demand for water. However, the rainfall is unreliable in Tarawa, as throughout the Gilberts, and underground water has to be utilized. The increasing demand has already caused the deterioration of the water lands, making it more saline. In Betio for example, water has become so brackish that it was declared unsafe to drink and a long water pipe was installed stretching from Bonriki to Betio. But if the present expansion rate continues this source will soon be exhausted(15).

Thus economic planners cannot ignore the role of health development. Equally those involved in health cannot stand by and let those engaged in economic development go their merry way and then comment on the consequences after the deed has been done. As Abel Smith and A. Leiserson pointed out in the first issue of <u>World Health Forum</u>:

> Social and Economic Planning should be seen as complementary, not competitive. The task of the health administrator and the economic planner is to work in cooperation for the mutual benefit and in the end for the well-being of the people they serve.

Though tourism has been used as an example in this instance it should not be seen as the only culprit because any inadequately planned economic venture can bring with it ramifications which have a disastrous consequence for the well-being of the people of a country. For instance, a hydro-electric scheme that may do damage to marine life can be no less guilty. Equally industrial development which pollutes not only the sea but the atmosphere can while earning profits for some bring health hazards for many. Unless carefully planned and closely monitored, development of the type Dr. Epeli Ha'ofa mentions in his work Corned Beef and Tapioka: A Report on the Food Distribution Systems of Tonga can be disadvantageous(16). He holds that though there is great demand for fresh fish in the main island of Tongatapu of the Kingdom of Tonga much of the catch that the Government obtains from deep-sea fishing instead of going to satisfy the needs of local people goes off to the canneries in Pago Pago (Western Samoa) and Levuka,(Fiji) for much needed foreign earnings. As a result Tongans continue to buy imported, frozen and canned meat and fish which are of an inferior quality compared to what they have exported for foreign exchange and someone else's nutritional needs.

Indeed the whole question of food production will need close study in a research project looking at the sectoral health in the South Pacific. Not merely the issue of nutrition but also other issues such as the availability of land, markets, methods of distribution as well as productivity will all have to be considered. Adequate emphasis nevertheless will have to be placed on the question of nutrition; this factor is looming large on the subject of health and development in the South Pacific. A recent survey in Fiji discovered that both Indian and Fijian children were under-weight and that this was the result of an insufficient intake of food of the right kind over a period of time. Many may not find this fact easy to digest given their mental pictures of island paradise or as a result of the large quantities of fruit and vegetables they might have seen on market-days in the South Pacific. The issue here is not of quantity but quality and a balanced diet. Since neither green vegetables nor meat seem to be in short supply it means that many are either ignorant about dietary matters or that they lack the means to purchase the right kinds of food. Of course, some also are susceptible to the propaganda that is read in the media regarding imported foods particularly those that come out of cans and bottles. In the Pacific it seems malnutrition is the result not of a lack of availability or even perhaps of maldistribution but a consequence of ignorance which can be removed through better education and dialogue between those involved with nutrition and the consumers. There is need to draw up a minimum diet for the Pacific Islanders engaged in various types of work because it is unlikely that some standard devised elsewhere will prove adequate. One ought not to ignore the fact that Pacific Islanders tend to be physically very big and that many of them do labour in very hot and humid tropical conditions doing physically strenuous work. It is an accepted fact that calorie intake and protein requirements vary with the size of the individual as well as with the type of employment. This hitherto seems not to have been noted by many who have talked about nutrition in the Pacific. Yet it is not only those in employment who are affected or afflicted, school children too are victims. Many a child who seems listless and inattentive in class is not infrequently in this condition because of a poor breakfast or no lunch. This point has apparently been noted in American Samoa where according to the Pacific Islands Year Book the Education Department provided 9000 lunches and 7250 breakfasts each day in 1976. While the other Pacific Islands states may not wish to emulate this plan completely they may nevertheless need to explore remedies based on what they may be able to afford or in fact be able to do for mal-nourished school children. Given the importance of education and poor performance in schools the relationship between the availability of food, parents' income, and school performance could be a very fruitful study. There is need for research in this area because a great deal is made by governments in some countries about the inability of some Pacific Islanders to cope with public examinations. In Fiji, comparisons tend to be drawn between the achievement of Indians on the one hand and the high failure rate of Fijians in public examinations at high school level or in tertiary institutions. While this is not meant to suggest that malnutrition is the sole cause of all difficulties in this case it may be one of several factors and if it is one of them then it is a very important one and the problem must be rectified. The answer to the problem of malnutrition lies not merely in producing more food but perhaps in producing more food locally and of the right kind because the point has been made by some writers that a poor diet has resulted from an increased consumption of imported food so argue Professor Terry McGee and his colleagues in their work on food distribution in the New Hebrides(17). For instance, they suggest, that important trace minerals are absent in meal rice and this inadequacy has to be supplemented from elsewhere. In their view a rapid increase in protein consumption in Papua New Guinea among the highlanders, people who previously relied very heavily on diets of carbohydrates, caused severe intestinal injuries, illnesses that tended to be fatal. They cite one authority as having reported that in Western Samoa shortage of both foreign and locally produced food was an important factor in the emergence of malnutrition and the decline in the birth weight of babies. Self-reliance on local food production is given prime significance in their recommendation because a decline in traditional food production could lead to a loss of skills which were previously used in the productive processes. This point is an important one because in the end Pacific Islands like other developing countries will have to depend on their own food production as it is very unlikely that the developed world would be able to supply them with sufficient quantities of quality food in case of shortage. Given the importance of nutrition in the developmental process and in the maintenance of health and given the fact that to understand its implications a variety of skills are needed this is an area where the skills of the social scientist and the medical practitioner can engage in fruitful interplay in research and the results will ensure a better quality of life for the people of the South Pacific.

Finally, a comment needs to be made about the role of Co-operatives because Pacific Islanders see this mode of economic operation as being in harmony with their traditional system and aspirations. For them this may be the means of humanizing capitalism and increasing production and distribution for the benefit of the Pacific Islanders themselves. While Co-operatives have been in the Pacific for some time now they still make the news usually when they fail rather than when some of them achieve something positive and beneficial for the people who have organised them. Dr. Roger Lawrence, in his report on the Island of Tamana in Kiribati has made the point that trading cooperatives seemed more effective than individuals working by themselves(18). In his view, people working together in a co-operative seem to show greater stability when it comes to resource access, labour availability and also motivation, or constancy of purpose, as he calls it. At this stage one needs to find out more both about why Co-operatives have failed and even more about those which have succeeded and then suggest ways in which they can be used in the existing mode of production to contribute to the betterment of the health of Pacific Islanders young and old.

This paper has explored a number of areas for research on this subject in the South Pacific, it may be best in conclusion to summarize these:

1. A general study of health and development of each South Pacific island state.

2. Studies of traditional child-rearing practices and their effect on the health of the child and the mother. If evidence is available some comparison might be made between the pre-European contact period and subsequently.

3. Studies of socio-economic impact of traditional medicine.

4. How to make educational systems more functional towards improving health in the community, both in rural and urban areas.

5. Studies of effective communication in the South Pacific, and how these can be utilised to improve child and maternal health. Ways to improve existing channels of communication between people and imposed systems of government now existing in the South Pacific.

6. Studies of alternative forms of government and administration, including decentralisation, in order to ensure involvement by the people in decision-making in sectors such as health. The intention is to find whether the delivery of health programmes can be made more effective.

7. The present state of the family in the South Pacific; its nature amidst social, economic and political changes including increasing urbanisation, growing and greater influence of outside educational and value systems, democratic

political organisation and changes in the role of traditional authority structures. How does the impact of these forces on the family affect its role regarding the maintenance of the health of not only the young and the aged but society as a whole.

8. The relationship between poverty and urban squatter settlements and the condition of health in these situations of poor housing and inadequate water and sanitation facilities.

9. Food production, local and foreign foods, socio-economic status and their consumption and the effect of these factors on the health of individuals and the community. Included in such a study will be the availability of land and credit as well as markets to individuals and groups. Since studies already exist on this topic regarding Fiji, Tonga and New Hebrides, their format and methodology might be extended to other island states, hitherto not examined.

10. Food, diet and educational achievement and performance of Pacific Islands in primary, secondary and tertiary institutions.

11. Case studies on nutrition and health in various island states.

FOOTNOTES

(1) Report of the Select Committee of Inquiry into the Health Services in Fiji. Parliamentary Paper,No.38 of 1979.

(2) Pacific Islands Year Book (13th Edition, 1978).

(3) Solomon Islands Year Book (1978).

(4) Nabiat Tafar, personal communication.

(5) Development Plan VIII, Vol.I.

(6) Paper presented to a seminar on Fourth World Children held at WHO Headquarters in Geneva in May 1981.

(7) 'Queen Salote Tupou III' in Noel Rutherford: Friendly Islands. A History of Tonga (O.U.P. 1977) p.207.

(8) Vanuatu (published by the Institute of Pacific Studies 1980) p. 143.

(9) ibid. p. 129.

(10) Fiji Parliamentary Paper, No. 17 of 1979, p. 29.

(11) E.K. Fisk: The Political Economy of Independent Fiji (Canberra 1970).

(12) Pacific Tourism As Islanders See It (Institute of Pacific Studies, Suva, 1981) p. 43.

(13) ibid. p. 85.

(14) ibid. p. 128.

(15) Vol. I, No. 1, 1979, p. 144.

(16) page 159.

(17) T.G. McGee et.al.: Food Distribution in the New Hebrides (Canberra 1980).

(18) R. Lawrence: Tamana Island Report, (Wellington, 1977).

CHAPTER THIRTEEN

LET US MAKE SURE EVERY NEW LIFE COUNTS

1. FUNDAMENTAL DEVELOPMENT FACTS THAT NOBODY KNOWS

The aim of this brief paper is to suggest a new approach to obtaining better data, especially relating to birth statistics, that will be helpful in health and development planning. It is a reaction to the present disastrous situation where, in many developing countries especially, the statistical base is so bad that it is very nearly impossible to be able to say anything with any scientific validity. Infant mortality rates, which have become one of the most important of all indicators, are often wildly inaccurate. There is a widespread underregistration of infant deaths for a wide number of reasons. It is an unpleasant, even tragic event. In some cultures, often because of the high level of infant mortality, a baby does not become a person for months, even years. An unintended, and unfortunate consequence of many birth control programmes has been that some babies (e.g. in large families) have been regarded as undesirable, and may easily become, therefore, unwanted.

2. POPULAR SUSPICIONS

More basically there is a fundamental suspicion by many people of the bureaucratic processes of which the registration of vital statistics and census-taking is a part. Many communities fear that information will be used against them in one way or another, for taxes, for military conscription and so on. These feelings are especially intense where there are elements of illegality as in the case of migrants.

3. BUREAUCRATIC FAULTS

It is not just people's fear that contributes to the bad situation. The processes of registration and census-taking are complex operations for which bureaucracies are often ill-equipped. The processing of census material may take so long that the information is out of date by the time it becomes available. Bureaucracies, often remote from communities (a separation increased by using computer technology), have often only a dim estimation of the accuracy of figures which is not helped by ill designed sample surveys. Because the figures are so bad there is encouragement for guestimates (which may more often reflect political contingencies rather than community realities) or the mathematical mumbo-jumbo that the number crunchers dream up.

4. CONSEQUENCES OF IGNORANCE

There are many other consequences of the ignorance of numbers and vital rates. Planning and targets based on per capita indicators of whatever kind (e.g. GNP per capita) are meaningless. Social development programmes reflecting statistical packages like the Physical Quality of Life Index (which combines infant mortality rates, expectation of life and literacy) reflect the mathematical consequence of weighting formulae rather than any grass roots realities. Interventions in health and other fields cannot be effective and there can be little evaluation of programmes. Since programmes are not effective, local opinion persits in a belief that figures are only used for dubious governmental purposes. There is no clear idea of benefit and therefore little motivation to help in the process of providing accurate statistics. There is, in short, yet another vicious circle which contributes to poverty and underdevelopment.

5. THE TOP-DOWN RESPONSE

The essential problem is then how to break the vicious circle. The standard response of the bureaucracy has been to try to obtain, by ever more force or cunning, more accurate statistics of the traditional kind. There may be attempts to tighten the laws and procedures on vital registration and introduce penalties for those who evade these regulations and the censuses. New techniques are devised which allow indirect estimates to be made for example of infant mortality rates working back from censuses. New sophisticated technology has been introduced, such as satellite remote sensing, even sideways radar, or there are proposals for rapid counts of bars of soap or what are considered as other important indicators. Monitoring, surveillance and evaluation are stepped up, but again it is doubtful whether, without the full co-operation of communities themselves, these exercises can be more substantial than catching shadows. Sticks are not usually as effective as carrots in making people do things.

6. REQUIREMENTS FOR A NEW APPROACH

What we are suggesting are new ideas which might ensure a more effective community participation. There are four essential requirements which need to be met:

(1) There needs to be a simple means of counting numbers of people and calculating infant mortality rates;

(2) This count needs to be quite comprehensive so that there is a baseline from which future planning can proceed and retrospective analysis can be made. This new kind of simple time sample, may well obviate some of the distortions and difficulties produced by conventional surveys like 'The World Fertility Survey';

(3) It needs to be a count which people in the community make themselves and is therefore information which is willingly divulged;

(4) To provide this information, there needs to be an expectation that there will be real benefits to individuals in the community. It should be made clear that the object is to count every new life in order to make every new life count.

7. BASIC STEPS

We are suggesting the following steps:

(i) The mothers be asked to record every new birth, every new life, and that initially at least, other information is kept to an absolute minimum (where possible birth weight could be included);

(ii) That this information is recorded in a very simple fashion, e.g. on a durable card which can be handed in to the local health worker, or to local institutions such as post offfices and cooperatives or put in a specially placed box or counting house, etc. The possibility of oral recording should be explored. The latter method might help to allay local suspicions. The new technology of oral data storage would fit in well with traditional concepts here;

(iii) The data collected could be integrated into the delivery of MCH services. Certainly the expectation should be that in return for helping in the campaign the mother would be offered MCH services and assistance, possibly appropriate food, housing or credit, so that both she and her child could be healthy and have access to other opportunities. It might be appropriate that when the mother or a family member does record the birth, they are given a book which outlines all the services available and how to get hold of them;

(iv) The recording of the birth would entitle the mother to an introduction to any other handouts or credits that were being offered. A credit card or coupon system could be used.

8. ORGANIZATION OF THE CAMPAIGN

Much of the success of the exercise would depend on the organization of a Campaign. The following features are suggested:

(i) The campaign should extend over a reasonably long period - say one year. Possibly the international agencies could designate a year for this purpose, but basically once the seed has been sown, the stimulus must come from the countries;

(ii) A good deal of publicity (and therefore investment) is needed as the campaign needs to be carefully prepared at the country level. The purposes should be widely advertised in the mass media. It might be appropriate to attempt to use local folk media to get the idea across. Certainly the motto needs to be widely displayed;

(iii) To accomplish the tasks an intersectoral committee ought to be set up - for all the sectors have needs for the kinds of information which the LET US COUNT EVERY NEW LIFE campaign will throw up, as well as being needed for the distribution of services that mothers will expect;

(iv) The committee should consult and co-opt at the very earliest stage the local communities so that they can be involved in planning the nuts and bolts part of the exercise - how the cards can be collected and particularly how mothers can obtain the benefits that will accrue to them as a reward for their co-operation, and how to prevent and control the conflicts and abuses that might arise;

(v) The committee needs to be not only governmental. It might be useful there to involve industry who could play a role in co-operating in any distrubtions of food, or technology for example, as well as advising on advertising. This might be a useful beginning for a public service role. It is most important that the mass media are involved since it is essential that the message is widely aired on radio and television and in the press.

9. IMMEDIATE TASKS

The following immediate tasks seem to be called for:

(i) The idea might be tried out on a pilot basis in areas of countries where there are already MCH services into which the 'Let us Count' proposals could plug in;

(ii) It would be best if these areas were in different regions, involving different socio-economic situations, so that there is a range of different experiences that can be drawn on to plan the major campaign;

(iii) This is intended to be basically a 'suck it and see' exercise, i.e. learning by experience. Nevertheless it would be very useful to have a summary of experience of similar type exercises, especially an analysis of the problems, pitfalls and possibilities. This may be a job the international agencies could do;

(iv) Certainly every effort should be made to utilize as quickly as possible, results and pointers from the 'Let us Count' campaign. This material should be fed as rapidly as possible into the Technical Co-operation between Developing Countries (TCDC) and similar systems.

Contributors

Addo, Herb
Institute of International Relations, University of West Indies, Port of Spain, Trinidad

Ali, Ahmed
Institute of Social and Administrative Studies, University of South Pacific, Suva, Fiji

Annandale, Viopapa
Health Department, Apia, Western Samoa

Ayalew, Solomon
Supreme Council of Planing, Addis Ababa, Ethiopia

Gunatilleke, Godfrey
Marga Institute, Colombi, Sri Lanka

Levi, Rula
Development Bank of Western Samoa, Apia, Western Samoa

Sapolu, Iuni
Health Department, Apia, Western Samoa

Yusof, Khairuddin
Dept. of Obstetrics and Gynaecology, University of Malaya, Kuala Lumpur, Malaysia

Participants in the Iketsetseng Series

Our participants come from over 20 countries, mostly in the third world, and there are equal numbers of men and women. They have included Herb Addo (Trinidad), Ahmed Ali (Fiji), Vio Annandale (Western Samoa), Solomon Ayalew (Ethiopia), François Breton (France), Bo Carlsson (Sweden), Nigel Cantwell (Switzerland), Cecilia Muñoz de Castillo (Colombia), Ihsan Dogramaci (Turkey), Edward Dommen (Switzerland), Shanti Ghosh (India), Francine de la Gorce (France), Godfrey Gunatilleke (Sri Lanka), Janal Hartouche (Lebanon), Jürgen Hartmann (Austria), Rula Levi (Western Samoa), Leah Levin (Great Britain), Michel Manciaux (France), Usha Naidu (India), Philista Onyango (Kenya), Else Øyen (Norway), David Pitt (New Zealand), M. Sainju (Nepal), Manthoua Seipobi (Lesotho), P. M. Shah (India), Göran Sterky (Sweden), Sjef Teuns (Netherlands), Soon Young Yoon (S. Korea), Khairrudin Yusof (Malaysia), Jerzy Zubrzycki (Australia).

Inevitably, there ist also a long list of people to thank in the production of any book — and especially so when a strong element of cooperation is involved, as was the case here. The contribution of many members of WHO's staff and members of different countries was indispensable and is gratefully acknowledged. Similarly, the secretariat of SIDA-SAREC (Sweden) provided an immense stimulus as well as the original funding for the project.

How Can You Participate and Help with the Iketsetseng Project?

- ○ Please send us your reactions.
- ○ Please suggest titles, or provide materials, for new issues. Please suggest modifications or alterations.
- ○ Please pass this on to a colleague, or put it in a library. Talk it about to your friends, on the radio, the bus or anywhere else. Tell the newspapers about it.
- ○ If you are a teacher, pass it on to students. Ask your students to write about their own experiences and what they consider to be necessary changes.
- ○ Please give us names to add to our network of those who would like to receive this and other issues.
- ○ Especially, please communicate these ideas to local people, ask for their ideas and reactions. Send us their views and stories, which illustrate the themes.
- ○ Tell us how these ideas can be translated into action at the local level.
- ○ Tell us how national or international organizations or others can help in this process.
- ○ Please send us titles of relevant publications that you would like to be included in an annotated bibliography. Tell us if you have trouble getting books and literature.
- ○ Send us any research proposals you have.
- ○ Please tell us if you can use a radio/cassette or film/television version of any of the Iketsetseng to help in the dialogue. Please tell us if any useful audio-visual materials already exist.

Please send all correspondence to:

Iketsetseng
c/o Defence for Children International
P. O. Box 92
CH-1226 Geneva-Thonex
Switzerland

WE LOOK FORWARD TO HEARING FROM *YOU*

Volumes in the Iketsetseng Series

1981 Child Labour: A Threat to Health and Development
Published by Defence for Children, P.O.Box 92, 1226 Geneva-Thônex, Switzerland

1982 The Poorest of the Richest: The Health and Welfare of the Excluded Child
Published by Defence for Children, Geneva

1982 War and Child Health
Published by the Geneva Peace Research Institute (GPRI), 41 rue de Zurich, Geneva, Switzerland

1982 Self-Reliance — The Future of Child Health and Development
Published by Mouton, Berlin, New York, Amsterdam

1983 Child Labour and Health in India
Published by The Tata Institute for the Social Sciences, Bombay, India

Bei Fragen zur Produktsicherheit wenden Sie sich bitte an:
If you have any questions regarding product safety,
please contact:

Walter de Gruyter GmbH
Genthiner Straße 13
10785 Berlin
productsafety@degruyterbrill.com